Dosage Calculations

made

Incredibly Easy!

TM

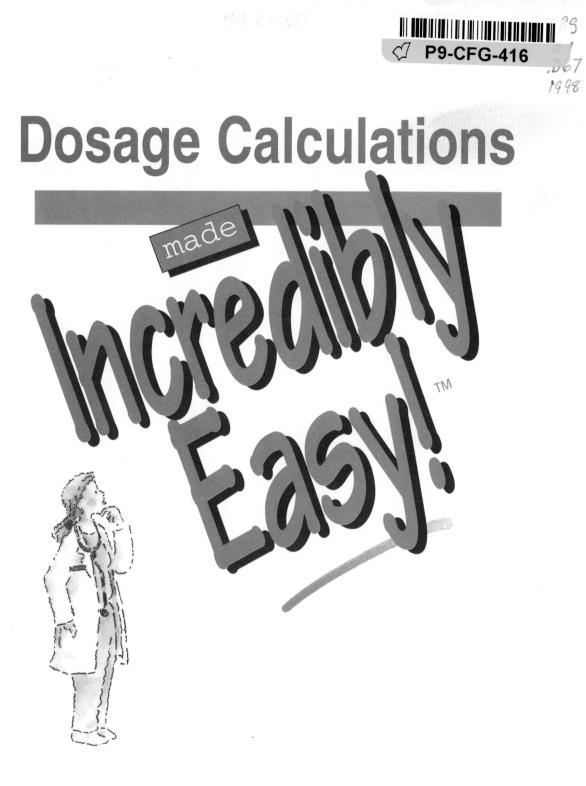

Springhouse Corporation
Springhouse, Pennsylvania

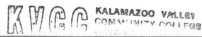

Staff

Executive Director
Matthew Cahill

Clinical Manager
Judith A. Shilling McCann, RN, MSN

Art Director
John Hubbard

Senior Editor
Michael Shaw

Clinical Editors
Mary Beth Morrell, RN, CCRN;
Ann M. Barrow, RN, MSN, CCRN
(project managers); Theresa P.
Fulginiti, RN, BSN, CEN;
Carla M. Roy, RN, BSN

Editors
Mary Lou Ambrose, Patricia Wittig

Copy Editors
Cynthia C. Breuninger (manager),
Mary T. Durkin, Brenna H. Mayer,
Karen C. Comerford

Designers
Arlene Putterman (associate art director),
Matie Patterson (assistant art director),
Mary Ludwicki (book designer)

Illustrators
Bot Roda, Jackie Facciolo

Typography
Diane Paluba (manager), Joyce Rossi
Biletz, Phyllis Marron, Valerie Rosenberger

Manufacturing
Deborah Meiris (director), T.A. Landis,
Otto Mezei

Production Coordinator
Margaret A. Rastiello

Editorial Assistants
Beverly Lane, Mary Madden

Indexer
Barbara Hodgson

Contents

Contributors and consultants

Lillian S. Brunner, RN, MSN, ScD
Nurse-Author and Consultant
Lancaster, Pa.

Bridget A. Haupt, PharmD
Director of Pharmacy
Children's Seashore House
Philadelphia

Catherine Nebe, RPh
Staff Pharmacist
Children's Seashore House
Philadelphia

Margaret R. Rateau, RN, MSN
Assistant Professor of Nursing
Kent State University, East Liverpool (Ohio)
Regional Campus

Nancy V. Runta, RN,C, BSN, CCRN
Medical-Surgical Staff Development
Educator
North Penn Hospital
Lansdale, Pa.

Maryann Summers, RN, MS
Nurse-Instructor
James Martin School for LPNs at Swenson
Skills Center
Philadelphia

David L. Wolff
Mathematics Teacher
Upper Dublin High School
Ft. Washington, Pa.
Associate Professor of Mathematics
Montgomery County Community College
Blue Bell, Pa.

Bonnie Zauderer, RN, MS, CNS
Assistant Professor of Clinical Nursing
University of Texas–Houston Health
Science Center
School of Nursing

Foreword

The focus of this book is a four-letter word that strikes fear in the hearts of too many nurses: Math. But let's face it: Numbers and nursing go together. Think of how many times you use numbers in the course of a working day: reading laboratory reports, transcribing orders, weighing patients, taking vital signs, recording intake and output and, last but not least, calculating drug dosages.

Among many people, math has an unfortunate reputation. Some people associate math with long, tortured equations written out across a blackboard and the horrid sound of squeaking chalk. Others think of math as a remote, abstract science. Still other people equate math with long, dull lists of figures in an accountant's journal.

For nurses, however, math is more than abstract reasoning or rote calculations. Nurses must apply mathematical concepts to real-world situations in which a patient's well-being or life itself may be at stake. That's why the clinical experts at Springhouse created a special math manual for nurses — one that's fun to use, entertaining, and so clear and concise that even the most math-phobic caregiver will enjoy and profit from using it.

The title of this book is *Dosage Calculations Made Incredibly Easy*. No doubt some of you reading this foreword are thinking like my friend in the left hand corner. Well, I challenge any and all of you to thumb through the following pages and see for yourselves. *Dosage Calculations Made Incredibly Easy* is fun as well as practical and informative.

To build your confidence, *Dosage Calculations Made Incredibly Easy* begins with a review of basics, including decimals, fractions, percentages, ratios, and proportions. Once you've mastered the fundamentals, the book walks you through hundreds of examples of interpreting drug orders and performing complex dosage calculations.

For example, you'll learn how to convert between measurement systems; how to analyze dosage calculation problems and set up proportions to solve them; how to determine infusion rates, flow rates, and drip rates for I.V. dosages; and how to solve special calculations for pediatric and critical-care drug dosages. Each calculation is written out step-by-step, with the rationale for each step explained in crystal-clear terms.

In addition to calculations, you'll find information on other vital aspects of dispensing drugs, such as deciphering difficult abbreviations and unclear

A dosage calculation book that's fun and entertaining? Yeah, right! Now I've heard everything!

handwriting, reading medication labels, selecting administration equipment, and more.

You'll also find many special features to enhance skills and strengthen understanding. Each chapter begins with an at-a-glance summary of key topics. Checklists on just about every page make it easy to spot the most important points. A *Quick quiz* at the end of each chapter helps you assess what you've learned. Special logos throughout each chapter alert you to essential information:

Before you give that drug contains urgent advice on how to avoid dangerous drug errors.

For math phobics only directs you to terrific hints, tips, and illustrations and encourages you to get over those "I hate math!" hurdles.

In a nutshell, *Dosage Calculations Made Incredibly Easy* will help you feel confident about administering drugs safely, reduce anxiety and frustration, and experience a sense of accomplishment as you master concepts and calculations in each chapter and progress toward more advanced skills. I recommend keeping a copy of it on your unit for quick reference.

When performing dosage calculations, only one goal is acceptable: No errors. *Dosage Calculations Made Incredibly Easy* will help you reach this goal. If it also helps you believe that strengthening math skills can be fun and fulfilling, that's okay, too.

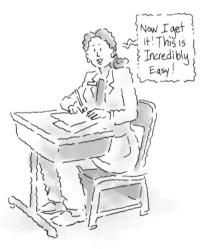

A special note for math phobics: If the sight of a complicated order or a long math equation makes you diaphoretic, relax! *Dosage Calculations Made Incredibly Easy* will cure your math phobia in 14 easy chapters.

Lillian S. Brunner, RN, MSN, ScD
Nurse-Author and Consultant

Part I

Math basics

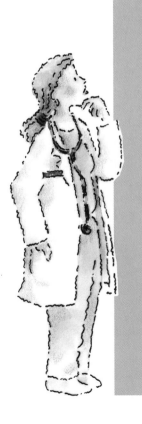

Fractions

Just the facts

In this chapter, you'll learn:

♦ what a fraction is

♦ different types of fractions you may use

♦ how to convert fractions, reduce them to their lowest terms, and find the lowest common denominator

♦ how to add, subtract, multiply, and divide fractions.

A look at fractions

A fraction represents the division of one number by another number. It's a mathematical expression for parts of a whole. (See *Parts of a whole*.)

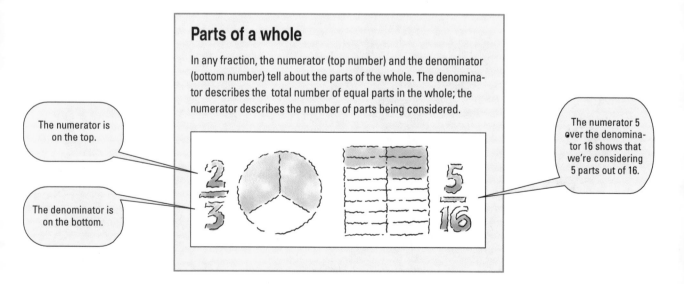

Parts of a whole

In any fraction, the numerator (top number) and the denominator (bottom number) tell about the parts of the whole. The denominator describes the total number of equal parts in the whole; the numerator describes the number of parts being considered.

The numerator is on the top.

The denominator is on the bottom.

The numerator 5 over the denominator 16 shows that we're considering 5 parts out of 16.

Getting to the bottom of it

The bottom number, or denominator, represents the total number of equal parts in the whole. The larger the denominator, the greater the number of equal parts. For example, in the fraction ³/₅, the denominator 5 indicates that the whole has been divided into five equal parts. In the fraction ⁷/₁₂, the denominator 12 indicates that the whole has been divided into 12 equal parts. So, as the denominator becomes larger, the size of the parts becomes smaller.

Staying on top of it

The top number, or numerator, signifies the number of parts of the whole being considered. For example, in the fraction ³/₅, only 3 of the 5 equal parts are being considered. In the fraction ⁷/₁₂, only 7 of the 12 equal parts are being considered.

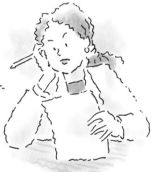

> **Memory jogger**
>
> To remember that the numerator is on top of the denominator, think of **ND** (N is first, then D), the initials of Notre Dame, the well-known university and home of the Fighting Irish.

Types of fractions

Fractions come in four types:
- common
- complex
- proper
- improper.

Common and complex

In a common fraction, such as ²/₃, both the numerator and denominator are whole numbers.

In a complex fraction, the numerator and denominator are fractions:

$$\frac{^2/_7}{^5/_{16}}$$

Proper and improper

In a proper fraction, such as ¼, the numerator is smaller than the denominator.

In an improper fraction, such as ⁸/₇ or 1¼, the numerator is larger than the denominator. In other words, it's "top heavy." An improper fraction represents a number that's greater than 1.

An improper fraction can also be expressed as a mixed number—a whole number and a fraction. Therefore, ⁸/₇ can be rewritten as:

$$1\tfrac{1}{7}$$

and $1\frac{1}{4}$ can be rewritten as:

$$2\frac{3}{4}$$

Working with fractions

Three mathematical techniques are commonly performed to manipulate fractions:
• converting mixed numbers to improper fractions and vice versa
• reducing fractions to their lowest terms
• finding the lowest common denominator.

Converting mixed numbers to improper fractions

To convert a mixed number to an improper fraction, do the following:

Multiply the denominator by the whole number.

Add the product of step 1 to the numerator (this gives you a new numerator).

Leave the denominator the same.

Three incredibly easy steps

For example, to convert the mixed number $5\frac{1}{3}$ to an improper fraction:

Multiply the denominator 3 by the whole number 5, for a total of 15.

Add 15 to the numerator 1, for a new numerator of 16.

The denominator remains the same. The improper fraction is $\frac{16}{3}$:

$$5\frac{1}{3} \text{ is } \frac{16}{3}$$

Encore!

In another example, to convert the mixed number $8\frac{4}{5}$ to an improper fraction:

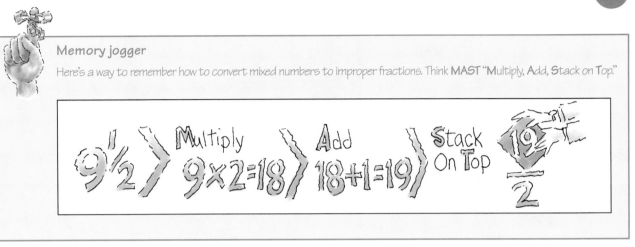

Memory jogger

Here's a way to remember how to convert mixed numbers to improper fractions. Think **MAST** "Multiply, Add, Stack on Top."

Multiply the denominator 5 by the whole number 8, for a total of 40.

Add 40 to the numerator 4, for a new numerator of 44.

Leave the denominator the same. The improper fraction is ⁴⁴⁄₅:

$$8\tfrac{4}{5} \text{ is } \frac{44}{5}$$

Putting it in reverse

At times, you may want to convert improper fractions back to mixed numbers.

To convert the improper fraction ¹⁶⁄₃ back to a mixed number:

Divide the numerator 16 by the denominator 3. You get 5 with 1 left over.

The 1 becomes the new numerator and the denominator stays the same.

The mixed number is 5⅓:

$$\frac{16}{3} \text{ is } 5\tfrac{1}{3}$$

One more time

To convert the improper fraction ⁴⁴⁄₅ back into a mixed number:

Divide the numerator 44 by the denominator 5. The answer is 8 with 4 left over.

✌ Place the 4 over the 5.

✌ The mixed number is 8⁴/₅.

$$\frac{44}{5} \text{ is } 8⅘$$

Reducing fractions to lowest terms

For simplicity's sake, a fraction should usually be reduced to its lowest terms; that is, to the smallest numbers possible in the numerator and denominator. To simplify a fraction, follow these steps:

✌ Determine the largest common divisor of the numerator and the denominator — the largest number that can be divided equally into both.

✌ Divide both the numerator and denominator by that number to reduce the fraction to its lowest terms.

> Reducing a fraction to its lowest terms will make my life simpler!

Example numero uno

To reduce the fraction ⁸/₁₀ to its lowest terms:

✌ The largest divisor that 8 and 10 have in common is 2.

✌ Divide the numerator and denominator by 2 to reduce the fraction to its lowest terms, or ⁴/₅.

$$\frac{8}{10} \text{ is } \frac{8 \div 2}{10 \div 2} \text{ is } \frac{4}{5}$$

Missed it? Watch again

Here are two more examples:

To reduce the fraction ⁷/₁₄ to its lowest terms:

✌ The number 7 is the largest divisor that 7 and 14 have in common.

✌ Divide the numerator and the denominator by 7 to reduce the fraction to its lowest terms, or ½. This fraction can't be reduced further.

$$\frac{7}{14} \text{ is } \frac{7 \div 7}{14 \div 7} \text{ is } \frac{1}{2}$$

To reduce the fraction ²/10 to its lowest terms:

 The number 2 is the largest divisor that 2 and 10 have in common.

Divide the numerator and the denominator by 2 to reduce the fraction to its lowest terms, or ⅕.

$$\frac{2}{10} \text{ is } \frac{2 \div 2}{10 \div 2} \text{ is } \frac{1}{5}$$

Finding a common denominator

One way to find a common denominator for a set of fractions is to multiply all the denominators. For example, to find a common denominator for the fractions ²/5 and ⁷/10, multiply the denominators — 5 and 10 — to get the multiplied common denominator, 50:

> Multiply the denominators . . .

$$\frac{2}{5} \quad \frac{7}{10}$$
$$\downarrow \quad \downarrow$$
$$5 \times 10 = 50$$

> . . . to find the multiplied common denominator.

To find the multiplied common denominator of the set of fractions ⅛, ¼, and ⅕, simply multiply all the denominators together to find the common denominator, 160:

$$8 \times 4 \times 5 = 160$$

Lowest common denominator

Unfortunately, multiplying all the denominators of a set of fractions won't always give you the lowest common denominator. The *lowest common denominator* or *least common multiple* — the smallest number that is a multiple of all the denominators in a set of fractions — is an important tool for working with fractions.

How low can you go?

One way to find the lowest common denominator for a set of fractions is to work with its prime factors. A *prime number* is a number that's evenly divisible only by 1 and itself. Some prime numbers are 2, 3, 5, and 7. *Prime factors* are prime numbers that can be divided into some part of a mathematical expression, in this case, the denominators in a set of fractions.

Prime factoring

Let's say you want to find the lowest common denominator for ⅛, ¼, and ⅕. Here's a useful technique, called *prime factoring*:
• Make a table with two headings: "Prime Factors" and "Denominators."
• Write the denominators 8, 4, and 5 over the top right columns.

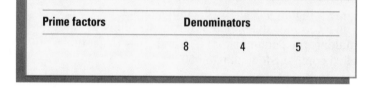

Prime factors	Denominators		
	8	4	5

• Divide the three denominators by the prime factors for each, starting with the smallest prime factor that divides into one of the denominators—in this case, 2. Write 2 in the left-hand column and divide it into the denominators. (Divide the denominator 8 by the prime factor 2 and write the answer, 4, in the column under the 8. Then divide the denominator 4 by the prime factor 2 and write the answer, 2, in the column under the denominator 4.)
• Bring down the numbers in the right-side columns that aren't evenly divisible by the prime factor in the left column. (In this case, the denominator 5 is not divisible by the prime factor 2 so just bring the 5 down.)

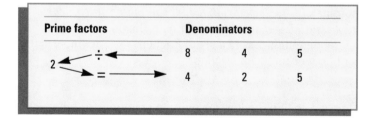

Prime factors	Denominators		
	8	4	5
2	4	2	5

• Repeat this process until the numbers in the bottom row can't be divided further. Here's what the table looks like:

Prime factors	Denominators		
	8	4	5
2	4	2	5
2	2	1	5
2	1	1	5

- Multiply the prime factors in the left column by the numbers in the bottom row. To say it with numbers:

$$2 \times 2 \times 2 \times 1 \times 1 \times 5 = 40$$

- The lowest common denominator for this set of fractions is 40.

Wow! Can you show me again?

O.K. Let's use prime factoring to find the lowest common denominator for ⅜ and ⅚. Create a table that lists the denominators horizontally. Find the prime factors.

Here's what the table looks like:

Prime factors	Denominators	
	8	6
2	4	3
2	2	3
2	1	3

- Then multiply the prime factors in the left column by the numbers in the bottom row:

$$2 \times 2 \times 2 \times 1 \times 3 = 24$$

Lowest common denominator

Once more, please

Now, use prime factoring to find the lowest common denominator for ⅓, ¼, and ½.

Here's the table:

Prime factors	Denominator		
	3	4	2
2	3	2	1
2	3	1	1

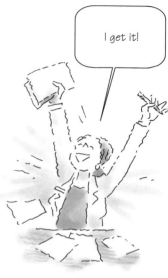

I get it!

Then multiply the prime factors in the left column by the numbers in the bottom row:

$$2 \times 2 \times 3 \times 1 \times 1 = 12$$

Lowest common denominator

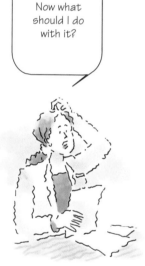

Now what should I do with it?

Converting fractions

Once you know the lowest common denominator of a set of fractions, you can *convert* the fractions so that all have the same denominator—the *lowest common denominator.*

One way to convert a set of fractions is to multiply each by 1 in the form of a fraction—that is, a fraction with the same number in the numerator and denominator. You find this fraction by taking the lowest common denominator and dividing it by the original denominator.

Here's what the formula looks like:

$$\frac{\text{original}}{\text{fraction}} \times \frac{\text{lowest common denominator} \div \text{original denominator}}{\text{lowest common denominator} \div \text{original denominator}}$$

This is how you convert a fraction using 1 in the form of a fraction.

Conversion excursion

Convert the set of fractions ⅛, ¼, and ⅕ so that each has the lowest common denominator. We already know that the lowest common denominator for this set of fractions is 40.

• Here's the conversion of the first fraction, ⅛, to ⁵⁄₄₀:

$$\frac{1}{8} = \frac{1}{8} \times \frac{40 \div 8}{40 \div 8} = \frac{1}{8} \times \frac{5}{5} = \frac{1 \times 5}{8 \times 5} = \frac{5}{40}$$

• Convert the next fraction, $\frac{1}{4}$, to $\frac{10}{40}$:

$$\frac{1}{4} = \frac{1}{4} \times \frac{40 \div 4}{40 \div 4} = \frac{1}{4} \times \frac{10}{10} = \frac{1 \times 10}{4 \times 10} = \frac{10}{40}$$

• Convert the last fraction in the set, $\frac{1}{5}$, to $\frac{8}{40}$:

$$\frac{1}{5} = \frac{1}{5} \times \frac{40 \div 5}{40 \div 5} = \frac{1}{5} \times \frac{8}{8} = \frac{1 \times 8}{5 \times 8} = \frac{8}{40}$$

Do it again

Here's how to convert $\frac{3}{8}$ and $\frac{5}{6}$ to fractions with the lowest common denominator, which is 24.
• Convert the first fraction, $\frac{3}{8}$, to $\frac{9}{24}$:

$$\frac{3}{8} = \frac{3}{8} \times \frac{24 \div 8}{24 \div 8} = \frac{3}{8} \times \frac{3}{3} = \frac{3 \times 3}{8 \times 3} = \frac{9}{24}$$

• Convert the other fraction, $\frac{5}{6}$, to $\frac{20}{24}$:

$$\frac{5}{6} = \frac{5}{6} \times \frac{24 \div 6}{24 \div 6} = \frac{5}{6} \times \frac{4}{4} = \frac{5 \times 4}{6 \times 4} = \frac{20}{24}$$

Once more

O.K. Convert $\frac{1}{3}$, $\frac{1}{4}$, and $\frac{1}{2}$ to fractions with the lowest common denominator, which is 12.
• Convert $\frac{1}{3}$ to $\frac{4}{12}$:

$$\frac{1}{3} = \frac{1}{3} \times \frac{12 \div 3}{12 \div 3} = \frac{1}{3} \times \frac{4}{4} = \frac{1 \times 4}{3 \times 4} = \frac{4}{12}$$

• Convert $\frac{1}{4}$ to $\frac{3}{12}$:

$$\frac{1}{4} = \frac{1}{4} \times \frac{12 \div 4}{12 \div 4} = \frac{1}{4} \times \frac{3}{3} = \frac{1 \times 3}{4 \times 3} = \frac{3}{12}$$

• Convert the last fraction, $\frac{1}{2}$, to $\frac{6}{12}$:

$$\frac{1}{2} = \frac{1}{2} \times \frac{12 \div 2}{12 \div 2} = \frac{1}{2} \times \frac{6}{6} = \frac{1 \times 6}{2 \times 6} = \frac{6}{12}$$

It's easy to convert a set of fractions!

Divide and conquer

You can also convert a set of fractions by using long division. To convert each fraction, follow these steps:

Divide the lowest common denominator by the original denominator.

Multiply the quotient by the original numerator to determine the new numerator.

Place the new numerator over the lowest common denominator.

Here's how to set up the conversion for each fraction:

$$\underset{\substack{\text{original} \\ \text{denominator}}}{}\overline{)\underset{\substack{\text{lowest common} \\ \text{denominator}}}{\overset{\text{quotient}}{}}} \times \underset{\text{numerator}}{\overset{\text{original}}{}} = \underset{\substack{\text{lowest common} \\ \text{denominator}}}{\text{new numerator}}$$

Set 'em up

Here's how to convert ⅜, ¼, and ⅖. The lowest common denominator is 40.

• The first fraction in the set, ⅜, is converted to ¹⁵/₄₀:

$$\frac{3}{8} = 8\overline{)40}^{\,5} \times 3 = \frac{15}{40}$$

• ¼ is converted to ¹⁰/₄₀:

$$\frac{1}{4} = 4\overline{)40}^{\,10} \times 1 = \frac{10}{40}$$

• The fraction ⅖ is converted to ¹⁶/₄₀:

$$\frac{2}{5} = 5\overline{)40}^{\,8} \times 2 = \frac{16}{40}$$

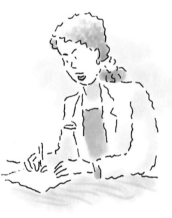

Amazing! Let's see that again

Here's how to convert ⅜ and ⅚. The lowest common denominator is 24.

• The fraction ⅜ is converted to ⁹/₂₄:

$$\frac{3}{8} = 8\overline{)24}^{\,3} \times 3 = \frac{9}{24}$$

• Convert ⅚ to ²⁰/₂₄:

$$\frac{5}{6} = 6\overline{)24}^{\,4} \times 5 = \frac{20}{24}$$

One last time

And here's how to convert ⅓, ¼, and ½. The lowest common denominator is 12.

- ⅓ is converted to ⁴/12:

$$\frac{1}{3} = 3\overline{)12}^{\,4} \times 1 = \frac{4}{12}$$

- ¼ is converted to ³/12:

$$\frac{1}{4} = 4\overline{)12}^{\,3} \times 1 = \frac{3}{12}$$

- ½ is converted to ⁶/12:

$$\frac{1}{2} = 2\overline{)12}^{\,6} \times 1 = \frac{6}{12}$$

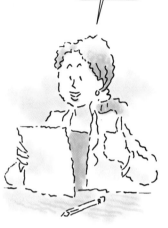

I can convert this set of fractions!

Comparing fraction size

Why are these calculations important? Because finding the lowest common denominator in a set of fractions allows you to compare the relative size of fractions. (See *Denominators can be deceptive.*) This concept is extremely useful for comparing the strengths of medications.

For math phobics only

Denominators can be deceptive

If you were hungry, would you rather have 1 slice from a pie that was cut into 4 slices, 8 slices, or 16 slices? You'd choose 4, of course, because the slices would be bigger. You can judge the size of fractions the same way. When the fractions all have the same numerators—in this case, ¼, ⅛, and ¹/16 — the fraction with the lowest or smallest denominator is the biggest one. Don't fall into the trap of thinking that the bigger the denominator, the bigger the fraction. Think in terms of a pie, as shown below.

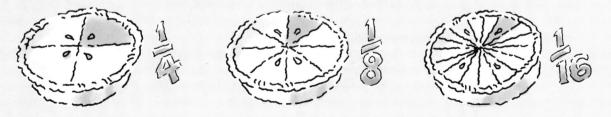

Oh, boy! A real world application

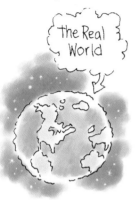

For example, suppose you want to compare the strengths of sublingual nitroglycerin tablets, which are available in $\frac{1}{100}$-grain, $\frac{1}{150}$-grain, and $\frac{1}{200}$-grain strengths. Follow these steps:

Using the prime factor method, first find the lowest common denominator for these three fractions. The table looks like this:

Prime factors	Denominators		
	100	150	200
2	50	75	100
2	25	75	50
5	5	15	10
5	1	3	2

Finally, multiply the prime factors in the left column and the numbers in the bottom row. In other words:

$$2 \times 2 \times 5 \times 5 \times 1 \times 3 \times 2 = 600$$

Lowest common denominator

Finding common ground

Next, convert all three fractions— $\frac{1}{100}$, $\frac{1}{150}$, and $\frac{1}{200}$— to new fractions with the lowest common denominator of 600. To do this, multiply each fraction by 1 in the form of a fraction (create this fraction by dividing the lowest common denominator by the original denominator). Here's the conversion:

• The fraction $\frac{1}{100}$ is converted to $\frac{6}{600}$:

$$\frac{1}{100} = \frac{1}{100} \times \frac{600 \div 100}{600 \div 100} = \frac{1}{100} \times \frac{6}{6} = \frac{1 \times 6}{100 \times 6} = \frac{6}{600}$$

• $\frac{1}{150}$ is converted to $\frac{4}{600}$:

$$\frac{1}{150} = \frac{1}{150} \times \frac{600 \div 150}{600 \div 150} = \frac{1}{150} \times \frac{4}{4} = \frac{1 \times 4}{150 \times 4} = \frac{4}{600}$$

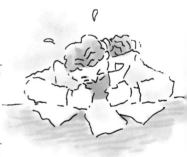

- The fraction $1/200$ is converted to $3/600$:

$$\frac{1}{200} = \frac{1}{200} \times \frac{600 \div 200}{600 \div 200} = \frac{1}{200} \times \frac{3}{3} = \frac{1 \times 3}{200 \times 3} = \frac{3}{600}$$

Comparing the three final fractions, you'll see that the $1/100$-grain nitroglycerin tablet offers the largest dose: $6/600$.

Another path

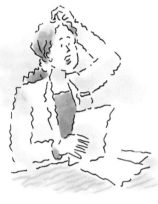

You can arrive at the same conclusion by dividing the lowest common denominator (600) by the denominator, multiplying the numerator by the number obtained, and placing the result over the lowest common denominator:

- The fraction $1/100$ is converted to $6/600$ this way:

$$\frac{1}{100} = 100\overline{)600} \times 1 = \frac{6}{600}$$

- $1/150$ is converted to $4/600$:

$$\frac{1}{150} = 150\overline{)600} \times 1 = \frac{4}{600}$$

- The fraction $1/200$ is converted to $3/600$:

$$\frac{1}{200} = 200\overline{)600} \times 1 = \frac{3}{600}$$

Fraction fact

When comparing fractions with common denominators, the fraction with the largest numerator is the largest number. In the set of fractions above, $6/600$ is the largest number.

The lowest common denominator does it again

The lowest common denominator also enables you to add and subtract fractions. Reducing fractions to their lowest terms and converting improper fractions to mixed numbers enables you to present the answers to addition, subtraction, multiplication, and division problems in a useful way.

Remember, whenever you perform these functions, always reduce the final answer to its lowest terms and, if it's an improper fraction, convert it to a mixed number.

Adding fractions

To add fractions, you first convert them to fractions with common denominators. (See *Comparing apples to apples*.)

It all adds up

Here's an example of adding fractions. Follow the steps below to add the fractions ⅐ and ⅓:
• First, find the lowest common denominator. Because the denominators in ⅐ and ⅓ are both prime numbers, multiply 7 by 3 to find the lowest common denominator, 21.
• Convert the fractions by multiplying each by 1 (in the form of a fraction) to yield fractions with the lowest common denominator:
• First convert ⅐ to ³⁄₂₁:

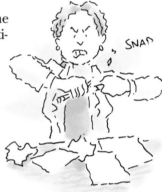
SNAP

$$\frac{1}{7} = \frac{1}{7} \times \frac{21 \div 7}{21 \div 7} = \frac{1}{7} \times \frac{3}{3} = \frac{1 \times 3}{7 \times 3} = \frac{3}{21}$$

• Next, convert ⅓ to ⁷⁄₂₁:

$$\frac{1}{3} = \frac{1}{3} \times \frac{21 \div 3}{21 \div 3} = \frac{1}{3} \times \frac{7}{7} = \frac{1 \times 7}{3 \times 7} = \frac{7}{21}$$

• Now, add the new fractions. To add fractions with a common denominator, add the numerators together and

---

Comparing apples to apples

When adding or subtracting fractions, don't forget to convert them to fractions with common denominators. This way, you'll be comparing apples to apples.

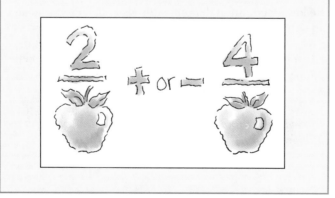

place the result over the common denominator. The resulting fraction is your answer. (Reduce it to its lowest terms, if possible.)

$$\frac{3}{21} + \frac{7}{21} = \frac{3+7}{21} = \frac{10}{21}$$

More addition

To add ½ and ⅕, follow these steps:

First, find the lowest common denominator. In this case, because the denominators 2 and 5 are both prime numbers, multiply 2 by 5 to find the lowest common denominator, 10.

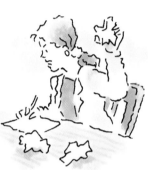

Convert the fractions by multiplying each by 1 (in the form of a fraction) to yield fractions with the lowest common denominator:

• Here's how you convert the fraction ½ to ⁵⁄₁₀:

$$\frac{1}{2} = \frac{1}{2} \times \frac{10 \div 2}{10 \div 2} = \frac{1}{2} \times \frac{5}{5} = \frac{1 \times 5}{2 \times 5} = \frac{5}{10}$$

• The fraction ⅕ is converted to ²⁄₁₀:

$$\frac{1}{5} = \frac{1}{5} \times \frac{10 \div 5}{10 \div 5} = \frac{1}{5} \times \frac{2}{2} = \frac{1 \times 2}{5 \times 2} = \frac{2}{10}$$

Now, add the converted fractions. To do this, add the numerators and place the result over the common denominator:

$$\frac{5}{10} + \frac{2}{10} = \frac{5+2}{10} = \frac{7}{10}$$

Additional addition

To add ⅗ and ⅔, follow these steps:

First, find the lowest common denominator; in this case, 15.

Convert the fractions by multiplying each by 1 (in the form of a fraction) to yield fractions with the lowest common denominator:

• Convert ⅗ to ⁹⁄₁₅:

$$\frac{3}{5} = \frac{3}{5} \times \frac{15 \div 5}{15 \div 5} = \frac{3}{5} \times \frac{3}{3} = \frac{3 \times 3}{5 \times 3} = \frac{9}{15}$$

- $^2/_3$ is converted to $^{10}/_{15}$:

$$\frac{2}{3} = \frac{2}{3} \times \frac{15 \div 3}{15 \div 3} = \frac{2}{3} \times \frac{5}{5} = \frac{2 \times 5}{3 \times 5} = \frac{10}{15}$$

To add the converted fractions, add the new numerators and place the result over the common denominator:

$$\frac{9}{15} + \frac{10}{15} = \frac{19}{15}$$

Reduce the fraction to its lowest terms:

$$\frac{19}{15} = 1\frac{4}{15}$$

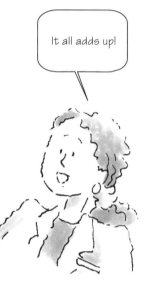

It all adds up!

Subtracting fractions

Like addition, subtraction requires converting fractions to terms with common denominators.

Fraction subtraction

Here's an example of how to subtract one fraction from another.

Follow the steps below to subtract $^1/_6$ from $^5/_{12}$:

First, find the lowest common denominator—in this case, 12. The fraction $^5/_{12}$ already has the lowest common denominator.

Convert the fraction $^1/_6$ to a fraction with the lowest common denominator. To do this, multiply the fraction by the number 1 (in the form of a fraction):

$$\frac{1}{6} = \frac{1}{6} \times \frac{12 \div 6}{12 \div 6} = \frac{1}{6} \times \frac{2}{2} = \frac{1 \times 2}{6 \times 2} = \frac{2}{12}$$

Now, subtract the numerators and place the result over the common denominator:

$$\frac{5}{12} - \frac{2}{12} = \frac{5 - 2}{12} = \frac{3}{12}$$

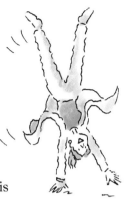

Reduce the fraction to its lowest terms, if possible. The resulting fraction is your answer:

$$\frac{3}{12} = \frac{1}{4}$$

A second subtraction

To subtract ⅑ from ⅚, follow these steps:

First, find the lowest common denominator; in this case, 18. (To find the lowest common denominator in this case, try prime factoring on your own.)

Convert the fractions to those with the lowest common denominator by multiplying each fraction by the number 1 (in the form of a fraction):

• Convert ⅚ to ¹⁵/₁₈:

$$\frac{5}{6} = \frac{5}{6} \times \frac{18 \div 6}{18 \div 6} = \frac{5}{6} \times \frac{3}{3} = \frac{5 \times 3}{6 \times 3} = \frac{15}{18}$$

• ⅑ is converted to ²/₁₈:

$$\frac{1}{9} = \frac{1}{9} \times \frac{18 \div 9}{18 \div 9} = \frac{1}{9} \times \frac{2}{2} = \frac{1 \times 2}{9 \times 2} = \frac{2}{18}$$

Then subtract the numerators and place the result over the common denominator. Reduce the fraction to its lowest terms, if possible. In this case, the fraction can't be reduced.

$$\frac{15}{18} - \frac{2}{18} = \frac{15 - 2}{18} = \frac{13}{18}$$

Additional subtraction

To subtract ¼ from ⅔, follow these steps:

First, find the lowest common denominator—in this case, 12.

Convert the fractions to those with the lowest common denominator by multiplying each fraction by the number 1 (in the form of a fraction):

- Convert ⅔ to ⁸⁄₁₂:

$$\frac{2}{3} = \frac{2}{3} \times \frac{12 \div 3}{12 \div 3} = \frac{2}{3} \times \frac{4}{4} = \frac{2 \times 4}{3 \times 4} = \frac{8}{12}$$

- Convert ¼ to ³⁄₁₂:

$$\frac{1}{4} = \frac{1}{4} \times \frac{12 \div 4}{12 \div 4} = \frac{1}{4} \times \frac{3}{3} = \frac{1 \times 3}{4 \times 3} = \frac{3}{12}$$

Subtract the numerators and place the result over the common denominator:

$$\frac{8}{12} - \frac{3}{12} = \frac{8 - 3}{12} = \frac{5}{12}$$

Multiplying fractions

Good news! You don't need to convert to common denominators. You simply need to multiply the numerators and denominators in turn.

For example, to multiply ⁴⁄₇ by ⅝, multiply the numerators 4 and 5 and the denominators 7 and 8 to get a new fraction. Here's the calculation:

- Set up the equation:

$$\frac{4}{7} \times \frac{5}{8}$$

- Multiply the numerators and multiply the denominators:

$$\frac{4 \times 5}{7 \times 8} = \frac{20}{56}$$

- Reduce the answer to its lowest terms:

$$\frac{5}{14}$$

Let's see it again

To multiply ⅚ by ⅓, multiply the numerators 5 and 1 and the denominators 6 and 3 to get the answer:

$$\frac{5}{6} \times \frac{1}{3} = \frac{5 \times 1}{6 \times 3} = \frac{5}{18}$$

Let's introduce a whole number

To multiply a fraction by a whole number, follow these simple steps:

• To multiply ⅑ by 4, first convert the whole number 4 to the fraction ⁴⁄1. The complete calculation looks like this:

$$\frac{1}{9} \times 4 = \frac{1}{9} \times \frac{4}{1} = \frac{1 \times 4}{9 \times 1} = \frac{4}{9}$$

Dividing fractions

In division (as in multiplication), you don't need to convert the fractions. Division problems are usually written as two fractions separated by a division sign. The first fraction is the number to be divided (the dividend), and the second fraction is the number doing the dividing (the divisor):

This fraction is the dividend.

$$\frac{5}{7} \div \frac{2}{3}$$

This fraction is the divisor.

To divide fractions, multiply the dividend by the divisor's reciprocal, or the inverted divisor. (See *Recipe for reciprocals*.)

Recipe for reciprocals

A reciprocal is an inverted fraction. It's used when dividing fractions.

A reciprocal is easy to make: Just flip the fraction like a hamburger.

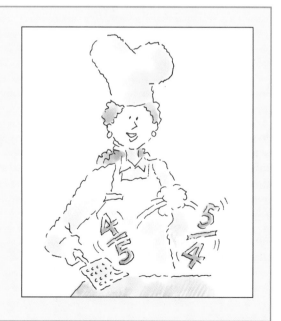

- To divide $5/7$ by $2/3$, first multiply the dividend ($5/7$) by the reciprocal of the divisor ($3/2$):

$$\frac{5}{7} \div \frac{2}{3} = \frac{5}{7} \times \frac{3}{2}$$

- Then complete the calculation and reduce the answer to its lowest terms:

$$= \frac{5 \times 3}{7 \times 2} = \frac{15}{14} = 1\frac{1}{14}$$

A part divided by a whole

To divide a fraction by a whole number, use the same principle.
- To divide $3/5$ by 2, first convert the whole number 2 to the fraction $2/1$.

$$\frac{3}{5} \div 2 = \frac{3}{5} \div \frac{2}{1}$$

- Then multiply the dividend ($3/5$) by the reciprocal of the divisor ($1/2$). Reduce the answer to its lowest terms:

$$= \frac{3}{5} \times \frac{1}{2}$$

$$= \frac{3 \times 1}{5 \times 2}$$

$$= \frac{3}{10}$$

In this case, the answer can't be further reduced.

Making life less complex

In complex fractions, the numerator and denominator are fractions themselves. Complex fractions can be simplified by following the rules for division of fractions. Think of the line separating the two fractions as a division sign. For example, follow the simple steps below to simplify the complex fraction:

$$\frac{1/3}{5/8}$$

👣 First, rewrite the complex fraction as a division problem:

$$\frac{\frac{1}{3}}{\frac{5}{8}} = \frac{1}{3} \div \frac{5}{8}$$

👣 Multiply the dividend (⅓) by the reciprocal of the divisor (⅝):

$$= \frac{1}{3} \times \frac{8}{5}$$

👣 Finally, complete the calculation:

$$= \frac{1 \times 8}{3 \times 5} = \frac{8}{15}$$

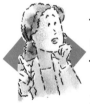

Quick quiz

1. ⅔ × 5⁄7 is:
   A.   14⁄15
   B.   10⁄21
   C.   7⁄5

Answer: B. To multiply two common fractions, multiply the numerators and then the denominators. The calculation looks like this:

$$\frac{2}{3} \times \frac{5}{7} = \frac{2 \times 5}{3 \times 7} = \frac{10}{21}$$

2.   In the fraction ⅘, the denominator is:
   A.   4
   B.   5
   C.   5⁄4

Answer: B. The denominator is the bottom number of a fraction. The numerator is the top number.

3. When you reduce the fraction ⁸⁄24 to its lowest terms, you get:
    A. ²⁄6
    B. ¾
    C. ⅓

Answer: C. Both the numerator and the denominator are divisible by 8, leaving the reduced fraction ⅓.

4. Which of the following is an improper fraction?
    A. ⁹⁄17
    B. 1½
    C. ⅓

Answer: B. An improper fraction has a numerator that's larger than the denominator.

5. When adding the fractions ½ and ⅓, you get:
    A. ⅚
    B. ³⁄6
    C. ⁵⁄20

Answer: A. To add ½ and ⅓, first find the common denominator, which is 6. Convert the fractions to ³⁄6 and ²⁄6. Then add the numerators and place the result over the common denominator. The calculation looks like this:

$$\frac{1}{2} + \frac{1}{3} = \frac{3}{6} + \frac{2}{6} = \frac{3+2}{6} = \frac{5}{6}$$

6. Of the following, the only prime number is:
    A. 4
    B. 5
    C. 6

Answer: B. The number 5 is a prime number because it can be divided only by itself and 1.

Scoring

☆☆☆   If you answered all six items correctly, wow! You're a number 1 math whiz (which is the same as a ²⁄2 math whiz and a ³⁄3 math whiz).

☆☆   If you answered four or five items correctly, fantastic! You're a freewheeling fraction fiend!

☆   If you answered fewer than four items correctly, stick with it! You've shown great derring-do in dealing with dividends and divisors.

Decimals and percentages

Just the facts

In this chapter, you'll learn:

♦ what decimals and percentages are

♦ how to add, subtract, multiply, divide, and round off decimal fractions

♦ how to convert common fractions to decimal fractions and vice versa

♦ how to convert percentages to decimal fractions and common fractions and vice versa

♦ how to solve percentage problems.

A look at decimals and percentages

For most people, decimals and percentages are a part of everyday life. Figuring a tip at a restaurant, balancing the checkbook, and interpreting the results of an election or a survey are just three ways people use decimals and percentages.

As a nurse, you also encounter decimals and percentages every day at work. The metric system, the most common system for measuring medications, is based on decimal numbers. You also use decimals and percentages when administering solutions, such as 0.9% saline solution, and drugs such as a 2.5% cream.

Here's what you need to know

To administer medications accurately and efficiently, you must understand what decimals and percentages are and how to work with them in common calculations. You also need to know how to convert from percentages to decimal fractions and common fractions, and then back to percentages. This chapter will sharpen your calculation skills and help you build confidence.

Deciphering decimals

A *decimal fraction* is a proper fraction in which the denominator is a power of 10, signified by a decimal point placed at the left of the numerator. An example of a decimal fraction is 0.2, which is the same as ²/10.

In a *decimal number*—for example, 2.25—the decimal point separates the whole number from the decimal fraction.

Look to the left...

Each number or place to the left of the decimal point represents a whole number that's a power of 10, starting with ones and working up to tens, hundreds, thousands, ten thousands, and so on.

...and then to the right

Each place to the right of the decimal point signifies a fraction whose denominator is a power of 10, starting with tenths and working up to hundredths, thousandths, ten

Know your places

Based on its relative position to the decimal point, each decimal place represents a power of 10 or a fraction whose denominator is a power of 10, as shown below.

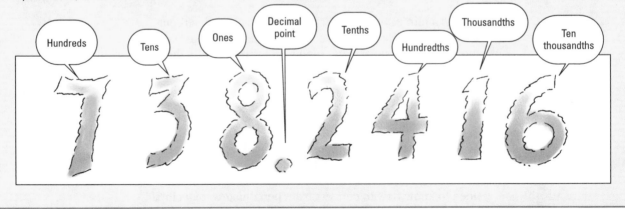

thousandths, and so on. (See *Know your places.*) When working as a nurse, you will rarely encounter decimal fractions beyond the thousandths place.

Getting to the point

When discussing money, people use the word *and* to signify the decimal point, for example, saying $5.20 as "5 dollars and 20 cents." However, when discussing decimal numbers in dosage calculations, use the word *point* to signify the decimal point. For example, say the number 5.2 as "5 point 2."

Zeroing in on zeros

Now that you've learned the basic terms used with decimal fractions, you're ready to review decimal calculations most often performed by nurses. But first, review these two important rules:
• After performing mathematical functions with decimal numbers, you may eliminate zeros to the right of the decimal point that don't appear before other numbers. (See *Zap those zeros.*)
• In other cases, you may wish to *add* zeros at the end of fractions (for example, as place holders). Deleting or adding zeros at the end of a decimal fraction does not change the value of the number.

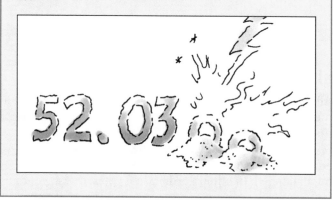

Zap those zeros

Are you solving a problem with decimal numbers? In most cases, you can delete all zeros to the right of the decimal point that don't appear before other numbers.

• When writing answers to mathematical calculations and specifying drug dosages, always put a zero in front of the decimal point if no other number appears there. This helps prevent errors. (See *Disappearing decimal alert.*)

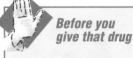

Adding and subtracting decimal fractions

Before adding and subtracting decimal fractions, line up the decimal points vertically to help you keep track of the decimal positions.

Placeholders please

To maintain column alignment, add zeros as placeholders in decimal fractions.

Here's how to use zeros to align the decimal fractions 2.61, 0.315, and 4.8 before adding:

$$
\begin{array}{r}
2.610 \\
0.315 \\
+4.800 \\
\hline
7.725
\end{array}
$$

Working it out

Here are two more examples of adding and subtracting decimal fractions. First, add 0.017, 4.8, and 1.22:

$$
\begin{array}{r}
0.017 \\
4.800 \\
+1.220 \\
\hline
6.037
\end{array}
$$

Next, subtract 0.05 from 4.726:

$$
\begin{array}{r}
4.726 \\
-0.050 \\
\hline
4.676
\end{array}
$$

Multiplying decimal fractions

Aligning the decimal points isn't necessary before doing a multiplication problem with decimal fractions. Just leave the decimal points in their original positions.

In the final product, the number of decimal places equals the sum of the decimal places in the numbers being multiplied. In other words, when you arrive at your an-

Disappearing decimal alert

Decimal points and zeros may be small items, but they're big deals on medication order sheets and administration records. When you get a drug order, study it closely. If a dose doesn't sound right, maybe a decimal point was left out or placed incorrectly.

For instance, an order that calls for ".*5* mg lorazepam I.V." may be mistaken for "*5* mg of lorazepam I.V." The correct way to write this order is by using a zero as a placeholder before the decimal point. The order would then become "0.5 mg lorazepam I.V."

swer, count up the decimal places starting from the right. Then place the decimal point. Here's how you'd multiply 2.7 and 0.81:

$$
\begin{array}{r}
2.70 \\
\times 0.81 \\
\hline
2.1870
\end{array}
$$

More multiplication

Here are two more examples of multiplying decimal fractions. First, multiply 1.423 and 8.59:

$$
\begin{array}{r}
1.423 \\
\times 8.59 \\
\hline
12.22357
\end{array}
$$

Next, multiply 42.1 and 0.376:

$$
\begin{array}{r}
42.1 \\
\times 0.376 \\
\hline
15.8296
\end{array}
$$

Dividing decimal fractions

When dividing decimal fractions, align the decimal points, but don't add zeros as placeholders. Begin by reviewing the parts of a division problem. (See *Let's call a divisor a divisor.*) *Remember: The number to be divided is the dividend, the number that does the dividing is the divisor, and the answer is the quotient.*

Whole-number divisors

Decimal point placement is easiest when the divisor is a whole number. Just place the decimal point in the quotient directly above the decimal point in the divisor, and then work the problem. For example, here's how to divide 4.68 by 2:

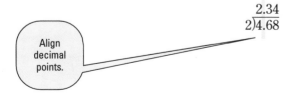

$$
\begin{array}{r}
2.34 \\
2\overline{)4.68}
\end{array}
$$

Align decimal points.

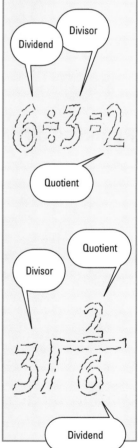

Let's call a divisor a divisor

Before you can divide numbers, you need to know what each part of a division problem is called. The division problem below can be written two different ways, but the terms remain the same:

Dividend
Divisor

6 ÷ 3 = 2

Quotient

Quotient

Divisor

3)6
2

Dividend

Decimal division double time

Here are two more examples of decimal point placement when the divisor is a whole number. First, divide 44.020 by 10:

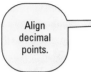

Align decimal points.

$$\frac{4.402}{10\overline{)44.020}}$$

Align decimal points.

Next, divide 9.093 by 3:

$$\frac{3.031}{3\overline{)9.093}}$$

Decimal-fraction divisors

Of course, not every divisor is a whole number—some are decimal fractions. Dividing one decimal fraction into another requires moving the decimal points in both the divisor and the dividend. (See *Dividing decimal fractions.*)

Rounding off decimal fractions

Most of the instruments and measuring devices a nurse uses measure accurately only to a tenth or, at most, to a hundredth. So you'll need to round off decimal fractions; that is, convert long fractions to those with fewer decimal places. (See *Remember rounding.*)

Overgrown decimals got you down?

To round off a decimal fraction, follow these steps:

☝ Suppose you want to round off the decimal fraction 0.4293. First, decide how many places to the right of the decimal point you want to keep. If you decide to round the number off to hundredths, you'll keep two places to the right of the decimal point and delete the rest (the 9 and the 3).

✌ Now, look at the first number that you've deleted—the number 9. Is this number 5 or greater than 5? Yes. So add 1 to the number in the hundredths place; that is, to the number 2. Your rounded off number is now 0.43.

🖖 Suppose the number that you delete is less than 5. Then don't add 1 to the number on the left. For example,

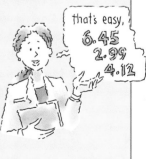

that's easy,
6.45
2.99
4.12

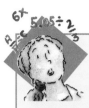

For math phobics only

Dividing decimal fractions

When dividing one decimal fraction by another, move the divisor's decimal point all the way to the right to convert it to a whole number. Move the dividend's decimal point the same number of places to the right. After completing the division problem, place the quotient's decimal point directly above the new decimal point in the dividend. The example below shows how to divide 10.45 by 2.6. The quotient is rounded to the nearest hundredth.

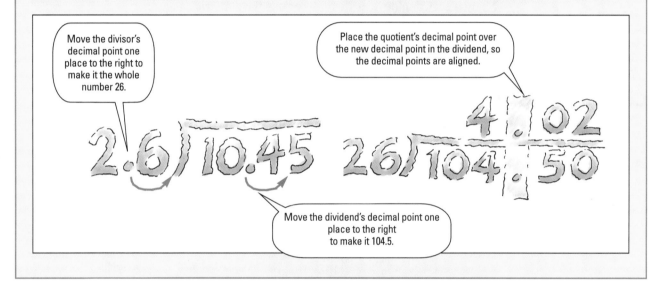

Move the divisor's decimal point one place to the right to make it the whole number 26.

Place the quotient's decimal point over the new decimal point in the dividend, so the decimal points are aligned.

Move the dividend's decimal point one place to the right to make it 104.5.

to round off 1.9085 to the nearest tenth, identify the number in the tenths position (9) and delete all the numbers to the right of it (0, 8, and 5). Because the number directly to the right of 9—the 0—is less than 5, the number 9 stays the same. The number 1.9085 rounded off to the nearest tenth is 1.9.

A practice round

Try rounding off 14.723 to the nearest hundredth:
• First, decide what number is in the hundredths place (2). Delete all the numbers to the right of it (only the number 3).
• Because 3 is lower than 5, you don't add 1 to the 2.
Thus, the rounded off number is 14.72.
        Now, round off 0.9875 to the nearest thousandth:

• The number in the thousandth place is 7. All numbers to the right of the 7—the 5—will be deleted.
• Because the number to be deleted is a 5, the 7 is rounded *up* to 8 (7+1). The rounded off number is therefore 0.988.

Converting fractions

Many measuring devices that nurses use have metric calibrations, so you'll often need to convert common fractions to decimal fractions. At times, you may also need to convert decimal fractions back into common fractions.

Converting common fractions to decimal fractions

Changing a common, proper fraction into a decimal fraction is simple. Just divide the numerator by the denominator. Add a zero as a placeholder to the left of the decimal point.

Commence converting

For example, here's how to convert $\frac{4}{10}$ to a decimal fraction:

$$\frac{4}{10} = 4 \div 10 = 10\overline{)4.0}^{\,0.4}$$

Keep on converting

Here are two more examples. First, convert $\frac{2}{5}$ to a decimal fraction:

$$\frac{2}{5} = 2 \div 5 = 5\overline{)2.0}^{\,0.4}$$

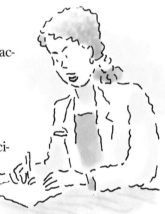

Next, convert $\frac{3}{8}$ to a decimal fraction:

$$\frac{3}{8} = 3 \div 8 = 8\overline{)3.000}^{\,0.375}$$

Converting mixed numbers to decimal fractions

How do you convert a mixed number to a decimal fraction? First, convert it to an improper fraction and then divide the numerator by the denominator, as shown above.

Mixing it up

Here's an example. To convert 4¾ to a decimal fraction, first convert the mixed number 4¾ to the improper fraction, ¹⁹⁄₄. Then divide 19 by 4 to find the decimal fraction:

$$4¾ = ¹⁹⁄₄ = 19 ÷ 4 = 4\overline{)19.00} \quad \frac{4.75}{}$$

Let's see that again

Here are two more calculations to try. First, convert 10⅞ to a decimal fraction:

$$10⅞ = ⁸⁷⁄₈ = 87 ÷ 8 = 8\overline{)87.00} \quad \frac{10.88}{}$$

Next, convert 1²⁄₉ to a decimal fraction:

$$1²⁄₉ = ¹¹⁄₉ = 11 ÷ 9 = 9\overline{)11.00} \quad \frac{1.22}{}$$

Converting decimal fractions to common fractions

To convert a decimal fraction to a common fraction, count the number of decimal places in the decimal fraction. This number reflects the number of zeros in the denominator of the common fraction.

For example, to convert the decimal fraction 0.33 into a common fraction, follow these steps:
• Count the number of decimal places in 0.33. There are two decimal places, so the denominator of its common fraction is 100, because 100 has two zeros.
• Remove the decimal point from 0.33, and use this number as the numerator. Reduce the fraction, if possible.

The calculation looks like this:

$$0.33 = \frac{33}{100}$$

This fraction can't be further reduced.

Practice, practice, practice

Try two more calculations. First, convert 0.413 to a common fraction. Here, the denominator is 1,000 because the decimal fraction (0.413) has three places after the decimal point.

The calculation looks like this:

$$0.413 = \frac{413}{1,000}$$

This fraction can't be further reduced.

Now convert 0.65 to a common fraction. The denominator is 100 because this decimal fraction has two places after the decimal point.

The calculation looks like this:

$$0.65 = \frac{65}{100} = \frac{13}{20}$$

Note that this fraction has been reduced to its lowest terms.

Converting decimal fractions to mixed numbers

Use the same method as above to convert a decimal fraction to a mixed number (or to an improper fraction).

Mixed up but methodical

For example, to convert 5.75 to a fraction, use 100 as the denominator because 5.75 has two decimal places. Then convert the fraction to a mixed number.

The calculation looks like this:

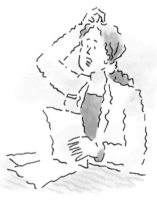

$$5.75 = \frac{575}{100} = 5\frac{75}{100} = 5¾$$

Note that this mixed number has been reduced to its lowest terms.

That was beautiful! Do it again

Below are two more sample calculations. First, convert 3.25 to a fraction. Use 100 as the denominator because 3.25 has two decimal places. Then convert the fraction to a mixed number.

The calculation looks like this:

$$3.25 = \frac{325}{100} = 3\,{}^{25}/_{100} = 3¼$$

Note that this mixed number has been reduced.

Let's see it once more

Convert 1.9 to a fraction. Use 10 as the denominator because 1.9 has one decimal place. Then convert the fraction to a mixed number.

The calculation looks like this:

$$1.9 = \frac{19}{10} = 1\%_{10}$$

Note that this mixed number can't be further reduced.

Understanding percentages

Percentages are another way to express fractions and numerical relationships. (See *A point about percents*.) The percent symbol may be used with a whole number such as 21%, a mixed number such as 34½%, a decimal number such as 0.9%, or a fraction such as ⅛%.

> ### A point about percents
>
> When you see "%", the percent sign, think "for every hundred." Why? Because percentage means any quantity stated as parts per hundred. In other words, 75% is actually ⁷⁵/₁₀₀, because the percent sign takes the place of the denominator 100.

From discounts to drug doses

You use percentages in everyday life when figuring department store discounts or restaurant tips. You also use them in nursing, when calculating solutions and drug doses. Because percentages are such an important part of your work, you must know how to convert easily from percentages to decimal fractions and common fractions and vice versa.

Converting percentages to decimals

To change a percentage to a decimal fraction, multiply the number in the percentage by $\frac{1}{100}$, or 0.01. For example, you would convert 84% and 35% to decimal fractions in this way:

$$84 \times 0.01 = 0.84$$

$$35 \times 0.01 = 0.35$$

Watch that decimal point

Make sure that you shift the decimal point in the right direction (to the left, when converting a percentage to a dec-

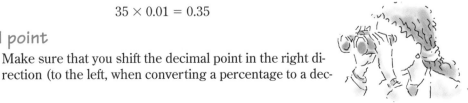

imal); otherwise you could calculate a drug dose incorrectly. (See *From percents to decimals [and back again]*.)

Converting percentages to common fractions

Suppose you want to convert 50% to a common fraction. To convert a percentage to a common fraction, follow these steps:

• First, remove the percent sign and put the decimal point two places to the left, creating the decimal fraction 0.50:

$$50\% = 0.50$$

• Next, convert 0.50 to a common fraction with a denominator that's a factor of 10. The result is $^{50}\!/_{100}$, because 0.50 has two decimal places:

$$0.50 = \frac{50}{100}$$

For math phobics only

From percents to decimals (and back again)

Though it seems like a harmless dot, a misplaced decimal point can cause a serious drug error. Study the examples below to see how to perform conversions quickly and accurately.

Jump to the left
To convert from a percentage to a decimal, remove the percent sign and move the decimal point two places to the *left*. Here's how:

$$97\% = 0.97$$

> Remove the percent sign. Move the decimal point two places to the left.

Jump to the right
To convert a decimal to a percentage, reverse the process. Move the decimal point two places to the *right*; add a zero as a placeholder, if necessary; and then add a percent sign. If the resulting percentage is a whole number, remove the decimal because it's understood. Here's how the calculation looks:

> Move the decimal point two places to the right and add a percent sign.

$$0.20 = 20\%$$

• Finally, reduce the fraction to its lowest terms, which is ½:

$$\frac{50}{100} = \frac{1}{2}$$

so,

$$50\% = \frac{1}{2}$$

Incredible! Do it again.

Here's another example. To convert 32.7% to a common fraction, remove the percent sign and put the decimal point two places to the left, creating the decimal fraction 0.327. Convert 0.327 to a common fraction using 1,000 as the denominator because 0.327 has three decimal places:

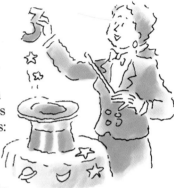

$$32.7\% = 0.327 = \frac{327}{1,000}$$

The result is ³²⁷/₁,₀₀₀, a fraction that's already reduced to its lowest terms.

Again?

Alright, one last example: To convert 20.05% to a common fraction, remove the percent sign and put the decimal point two places to the left, creating the decimal fraction 0.2005. Use 10,000 as the denominator because 0.2005 has four decimal places:

$$20.05\% = 0.2005 = \frac{2,005}{10,000} = \frac{401}{2,000}$$

The result is ²,⁰⁰⁵/₁₀,₀₀₀, which becomes ⁴⁰¹/₂,₀₀₀ when reduced.

Converting common fractions to percentages

Converting a common fraction to a percentage involves two simple steps. Suppose you want to convert ⅖ to a decimal. First, divide the numerator 2 by the denominator 5. You can do this by hand or use a calculator. (See *Thank heaven for calculators,* page 38.)

The calculation looks like this:

$$\frac{2}{5} = 2 \div 5 = 5\overline{)2.0}^{\,0.4}$$

Next, convert the decimal fraction to a percentage by moving the decimal point two places to the right (you'll need to add a zero as a placeholder), and then adding the percent sign. Here's what the calculation looks like:

$$0.40 = 40\%$$

Practice, practice, practice

Here's a second example. To convert ⅓ to a percentage, create a decimal fraction by dividing 1 by 3. Round off the quotient to two decimal places:

$$\frac{1}{3} = 1 \div 3 = 0.333 = 0.33$$

Then convert the decimal fraction to a percentage by moving the decimal point two places to the right and adding the percent sign:

$$0.33 = 33\%$$

Once more to be sure

Here's a third example. To convert ⅜ to a percentage, create a decimal fraction by dividing 3 by 8:

$$\frac{3}{8} = 3 \div 8 = 0.375$$

Thank heaven for calculators

A calculator can simplify converting a common fraction to a decimal fraction. For example, to convert a mixed number like 2⅘ to a decimal fraction, first convert it to the improper fraction ¹⁴⁄₅. Then follow these steps on the calculator:

1. Enter the numerator 14
2. Press ÷
3. Enter the denominator 5
4. Press = to obtain the converted number—2.8

Then convert the decimal fraction to a percentage by moving the decimal point two places to the right and adding the percent sign. The result is:

$$0.375 = 37.5\%$$

Solving percentage problems

Solving percentage problems involves three different types of calculations. They are:
• finding a percent of a number
• finding what percent one number is of another
• finding a number when a percentage of it is known.
    You'll have an easier time solving these calculations if you follow a few simple guidelines. (See *Percentage problems: Watch the wording*.)

Finding a percent of a number

The question "What is 40% of 200?" is an example of the first type of calculation. To solve it, change the word *of* to a multiplication sign. This gives you:

$$40\% \times 200 = ?$$

Next, convert 40% to a decimal fraction by removing the percent sign and moving the decimal point two places to the left. This gives you:

$$40\% = 0.40$$

Then multiply the two numbers to get the answer, 80:

$$0.40 \times 200 = 80$$

40% of 200 is 80.

Practice time (again)

Now, try solving the problem, "What is 5% of 150?" First, restate it as a multiplication problem:

$$5\% \times 150 = ?$$

Next, convert the 5% to the decimal fraction 0.05:

$$5\% = 0.05$$

Then multiply the two numbers to get the answer, 7.5:

$$0.05 \times 150 = 7.5$$

5% of 150 is 7.5.

Therefore, 7.5 is 5% of 150.

More practice (and you thought the piano was rough)

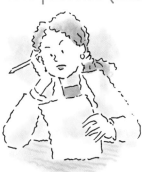

Here's one more example: "What is 7% of 300?" First, re-state the question as a multiplication problem:

$$7\% \times 300 = ?$$

Convert 7% to the decimal fraction 0.07:

$$7\% = 0.07$$

Then multiply the two numbers to get the answer, 21:

$$0.07 \times 300 = 21$$

21 is 7% of 300.

Finding what percent one number is of another

The question "10 is what percent of 200?" is an example of this type of calculation. To solve it, restate the question as a division problem, with the number 10 as the dividend and the number 200 as the divisor. Here's how the calculation looks so far:

$$200 \overline{)10.00} \quad 0.05$$

Now, move the decimal point in the quotient two places to the right, and add a percent sign:

$$0.05 = 5\%$$

10 is 5% of 200.

Again (with a twist)

This type of problem also can be expressed in this way: "What percent of 28 is 14?" To solve it, restate the question as a division problem by making 28 the divisor and 14 the dividend:

$$\frac{0.50}{28\overline{)14.00}}$$

Then move the decimal point two places to the right, and add a percent sign:

$$0.50 = 50\%$$

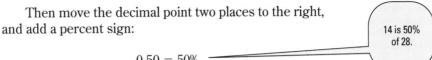

14 is 50% of 28.

One more time

Here's one last problem: "What percent of 30 is 6?" First, restate the question as a division problem by making 30 the divisor and 6 the dividend:

$$\frac{0.20}{30\overline{)6.00}}$$

Move the decimal point two places to the right, and add a percent sign:

$$0.20 = 20\%$$

6 is 20% of 30.

They don't all work out that neatly

Sometimes, when determining what percent one number is of another number, the divisor won't always divide exactly into the dividend. In these cases, state the quotient as a mixed number by turning the remainder—the undivided part of the quotient—into a common fraction.

Here's how to do this using the problem, "3 is what percent of 11?"

Restate the question as a division problem, making 11 the divisor and 3 the dividend. Work out the quotient to two places; then take the remainder 3 and make it the numerator of a fraction with the divisor 11 as the denominator.

Here's what the calculation looks like:

$$
\begin{array}{r}
0.27 \text{ and } {}^{3}\!/_{11} \\
11\overline{)3.00} \\
2\,2 \\
\hline
80 \\
77 \\
\hline
3
\end{array}
$$

Move the decimal point in the quotient two places to

the right, and add a percent sign. (The remaining fraction, $3/11$, is placed to the left of the percent sign.)

$$0.27 \text{ and } 3/11 = 27 \, 3/11 \%$$

Practice time

Let's try a second problem: "5 is what percent of 22?"

Restate the question as a division problem, leaving the remainder after two places as a common fraction:

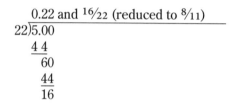

$$
\begin{array}{r}
0.22 \text{ and } 16/22 \text{ (reduced to } 8/11) \\
22\overline{)5.00} \\
4\,4 \\
\hline
60 \\
44 \\
\hline
16
\end{array}
$$

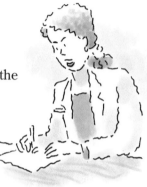

Move the decimal point in the quotient two places to the right, and add a percent sign:

$$0.22\,8/11 = 22\,8/11\%$$

Just can't get enough of those mixed number quotients

Here's the last example: "13 is what percent of 45?" Restate the question as a division problem, leaving the remainder after two places as a common fraction:

$$
\begin{array}{r}
0.28 \text{ and } 40/45 \text{ (reduced to } 8/9) \\
45\overline{)13.00} \\
9\,0 \\
\hline
4\,00 \\
3\,60 \\
\hline
40
\end{array}
$$

Move the decimal point in the quotient two places to the right, and add a percent sign:

$$0.28\,8/9 = 28\,8/9\%$$

Finding a number when you know a percentage of it

The third type of problem, finding a number when you know a percentage of it, also requires division. For example, consider the following question, "70% of what number is 7?" Here's how to do this calculation:

First, convert 70% into a decimal fraction by removing the percent sign and moving the decimal point two places to the left:

$$70\% = 0.70$$

Next, divide 7 by 0.70. Move the decimal point two places to the right in both the divisor (to make it a whole number) and the dividend. The quotient is 10:

$$0.70\overline{)7.00} \quad \begin{array}{c} 10. \end{array}$$

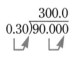

70% of 10 is 7.

Practice time

Now try the problem "30% of what number is 90?" To solve it, convert 30% to a decimal fraction by removing the percent sign and moving the decimal point two places to the left:

$$30\% = 0.30$$

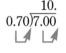

Then divide 90 by 0.30. Move the decimal point two places to the right in both the divisor (to make it a whole number) and the dividend. The quotient is 300.

$$0.30\overline{)90.000} \quad \begin{array}{c} 300.0 \end{array}$$

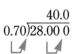

30% of 300 is 90.

Now you're getting the hang of it

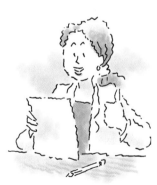

Here's a third example: "70% of what number is 28?" To solve this problem, convert 70% to a decimal fraction by removing the percent sign and moving the decimal point two places to the left:

$$70\% = 0.70$$

Then divide 28 by 0.70. Move the decimal point two places to the right in both the divisor (to make it a whole number) and the dividend. The quotient is 40:

$$0.70\overline{)28.00\,0} \quad \begin{array}{c} 40.0 \end{array}$$

70% of 40 is 28.

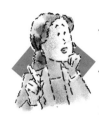

Quick quiz

1. 16% of 79 is:
   A. 0.20
   B. 4.16
   C. 12.64

Answer: C. To solve this, restate the question as a multiplication problem. Convert 16% to a decimal fraction by removing the percent sign and moving the decimal point two places to the left. The decimal fraction is 0.16. Then multiply 0.16 by 79.

2. The decimal fraction 1.9 divided by 3.2 yields:
   A. 0.59
   B. 1.5
   C. 10.55

Answer: A. To solve this, move the decimal points of both the divisor and the dividend one place to the right before dividing. Place the quotient's decimal point over the new decimal point in the dividend.

3. When 10.2467 is rounded off to the nearest hundredth, it becomes:
   A. 10.247
   B. 10.24
   C. 10.25

Answer: C. The number 4 is in the hundredths place. Look at the number to the right of it, which is 6. Six is greater than 5, so add 1 to 4 to round off the number.

4. Subtracting 0.003 from 2.5 yields:
   A. 0.2497
   B 2.497
   C 24.97

Answer: B. This answer was obtained by vertically aligning the decimal points and using zeros as placeholders before subtracting.

5. In the decimal fraction 1.2058, the number in the tenths place is:
   A. 2
   B. 0
   C. 1

Answer: A. The tenths place is to the immediate right of the decimal point.

6. Multiplying 4.9 by 10.203 yields the product:
- A. 49.9947
- B. 49994.7
- C. 0.499947

Answer: A. When multiplying, the number of decimal places in the final product equals the sum of the decimal places in the numbers being multiplied. Count the decimal places starting from the right, and place the decimal point there.

7. When the decimal fraction 0.75 is converted to a common fraction, the result is:
- A. $.75/100$
- B. $75/100$
- C. $7.5/100$

Answer: B. By moving the decimal point two places to the right and using 100 as the denominator, you obtain the correct answer. The fraction can be reduced to ¾.

8. When 3% is converted to a decimal fraction, it becomes:
- A. 0.03
- B. 0.30
- C. 3.0

Answer: A. Remove the percent sign and move the decimal point two places to the left.

9. When the decimal fraction 0.019 is converted to a percentage, it becomes:
- A. 0.19%
- B. 19%
- C. 1.9%

Answer: C. Move the decimal point two places to the right and add a percent sign.

10. Converting the common fraction ⅛ to a percentage yields:
- A. 12.5%
- B. 8%
- C. ⅛%

Answer: A. To obtain 12.5, divide 1 by 8, and then convert the answer to a percentage by moving the decimal point two places to the right.

Scoring

☆☆☆   If you answered all 10 items correctly, that's 100% (or $^{10}/_{10}$ or, if you prefer decimal fractions, 1.00).

☆☆   If you answered seven to nine correctly, excellent! As they say, $^{7}/_{10}$ to $^{9}/_{10}$ ain't bad.

☆   If you answered fewer than seven correctly, here's what to do: Subtract the number you got right from ten and add the result back to your score. Now you've got 100%. Reward yourself with a new calculator!

Ratios, fractions, proportions, and solving for *X*

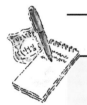

Just the facts

In this chapter, you'll learn:

♦ the definition of ratios and proportions

♦ how to set up proportions using ratios and fractions

♦ how to solve for *X* in an equation

♦ how ratios, proportions, and solving for *X* relate to dosage calculation.

A look at numerical relationships

Ratios, fractions, and proportions describe the relationships between numbers. Ratios use a colon between the numbers in the relationship, as in 4 : 9. Fractions use a slash between numbers in the relationship, as in ⁴⁄9.

Proportions are statements of equality between two ratios. For example, to show that 4:9 is equal to 8:18, you'd write:

$$4 : 9 :: 8 : 18$$

or

$$\frac{4}{9} = \frac{8}{18}$$

Three major problem solvers

When calculating dosages, you'll use ratios, fractions, and proportions frequently. You'll also use them to solve many other related problems, such as calculating I.V. infusion rates, converting weights between systems of measurement, and in specialty settings such as performing oxygenation and hemodynamic calculations. But before you can put ratios, fractions, and proportions to use, you need to know how to develop and express them appropriately.

Ratios and fractions

Ratios and fractions are numerical ways to compare items.

Dare to compare

If 100 syringes come in 1 box, then the number of syringes compared to boxes is 100 to 1. This can be written as the ratio 100 : 1 or as the fraction $^{100}/_1$.

On the other hand, the number of boxes to syringes would be 1 : 100 or the fraction 1/100, so pay attention to which item is mentioned first.

Here are two more examples:

If a hospital's critical care area requires 1 registered nurse for every 2 patients, then the relationship of registered nurses to patients is 1 to 2. You can express this with the ratio 1 : 2 or with the fraction ½.

Or suppose a vial has 8 mg of a drug in 1 ml of solution. By using a ratio, you can express this as 8 mg : 1 ml. By using a fraction, you can describe it as 8 mg/1 ml.

Proportions

A proportion is a set of equal ratios or fractions. Any proportion that's expressed as two ratios also can be expressed as two fractions.

Using ratios in proportions

When using ratios in a proportion, separate them with double colons. Double colons represent equality between the two ratios.

For example, if the ratio of syringes to boxes is 100 : 1, then 200 syringes are provided in 2 boxes. This proportion can be written as:

100 syringes : 1 box :: 200 syringes : 2 boxes

or

100 : 1 :: 200 : 2

Proportion practice

Here's another example. If the critical care area has 1 nurse for every 2 patients, you can express this as the ratio 1 : 2. You also can say that this equals a ratio of 3 nurses for every 6 patients. In a proportion, you can express this relationship with ratios as follows:

1 nurse : 2 patients :: 3 nurses : 6 patients

or

$$1 : 2 :: 3 : 6$$

More proportion practice

Now, suppose you have a vial that contains 8 mg of a drug in 1 ml of a solution. You can state this as the ratio 8 mg : 1 ml, which equals 16 mg : 2 ml. This proportion can be expressed with ratios as follows:

8 mg : 1 ml :: 16 mg : 2 ml

or

$$8 : 1 :: 16 : 2$$

Using fractions in proportions

Any proportion that can be expressed with ratios also can be expressed with fractions. Here's how to do this using the previous examples.

If 100 syringes come in a box, this means that 200 syringes come in 2 boxes. Using fractions, you can write this proportion as:

$$\frac{100 \text{ syringes}}{1 \text{ box}} = \frac{200 \text{ syringes}}{2 \text{ boxes}}$$

or

$$\frac{100}{1} = \frac{200}{2}$$

Fraction action

If the critical care area has 1 nurse for every 2 patients, this means that it has 3 nurses for every 6 patients. Using fractions, you can express this relationship as:

$$\frac{1 \text{ nurse}}{2 \text{ patients}} = \frac{3 \text{ nurses}}{6 \text{ patients}}$$

or

$$\frac{1}{2} = \frac{3}{6}$$

Proportion-style vial

If a vial has 8 mg of a drug in 1 ml, this means it has 16 mg in 2 ml. This proportion can be expressed with fractions as:

$$\frac{8 \text{ mg}}{1 \text{ ml}} = \frac{16 \text{ mg}}{2 \text{ ml}}$$

or

$$\frac{8}{1} = \frac{16}{2}$$

Solving for *X*

We know that a proportion is a set of two equal ratios or fractions. But what if one ratio or fraction is incomplete? In this case, *the unknown part of the ratio or fraction is represented by X.* You can solve for *X* to determine the value of the unknown quantity. (See *An explanation of X.*)

Solving common-fraction equations

The method used in solving common-fraction equations forms the basis for solving other types of simple equations to find the value of *X*. For example, here's how to solve the common-fraction equation:

$$X = \frac{1}{5} \times \frac{3}{9}$$

- Multiply the numerators:

$$1 \times 3 = 3$$

- Multiply the denominators:

$$5 \times 9 = 45$$

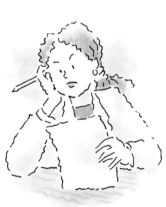

- Restate the equation with this new information:

$$X = \frac{1 \times 3}{5 \times 9} = \frac{3}{45}$$

- Reduce the fraction by dividing the numerator and denominator by the lowest common denominator (3), to find that $X = \frac{1}{15}$.

$$X = \frac{3 \div 3}{45 \div 3} = \frac{1}{15}$$

- Most dosage calculations require your answer to be in decimal form. So convert ¹⁄15 to a decimal fraction by dividing the numerator by the denominator. Round the answer off to the nearest hundredth. The final result is $X = 0.07$.

$$X = \frac{1}{15} = 1 \div 15 = 0.07$$

An "*X*-ample"

Now, solve for *X* in the equation:

$$X = \frac{2}{3} \times \frac{5}{8}$$

- Multiply the numerators:

$$2 \times 5 = 10$$

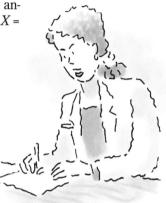

What does it all mean?

An explanation of *X*

Being able to find the value of *X* is vital in dosage calculations. For example, suppose a doctor orders a drug for your patient, but the drug isn't available in the correct strength. How do you decide on the right amount of drug to administer?

Here's how

Suppose you receive an order to administer 0.1 mg of epinephrine S.C., but the only epinephrine on hand is a 1-ml ampule that contains 1 mg of epinephrine. To calculate the volume for injection, state the problem in a proportion:

$$1 \text{ mg} : 1 \text{ ml} :: 0.1 \text{ mg} : X \text{ ml}$$

Rewrite the problem as an equation by applying the principle that the product of the means (numbers in the middle of the proportion) equals the product of the extremes (numbers at the end of the proportion).

$$1 \text{ ml} \times 0.1 \text{ mg} = 1 \text{ mg} \times X \text{ ml}$$

Solve for *X* by dividing both sides of the equation by the known value that appears on the same side of the equation as the unknown value *X*. Then cancel out units that appear in the numerator and denominator. (This isolates *X* on one side of the equation.)

$$\frac{1 \text{ ml} \times 0.1 \cancel{\text{ mg}}}{1 \cancel{\text{ mg}}} = \frac{\cancel{1 \text{ mg}} \times X \text{ ml}}{1 \cancel{\text{ mg}}}$$

$$X = 0.1 \text{ ml}$$

- Multiply the denominators:

$$3 \times 8 = 24$$

- Restate the equation with this new information:

$$X = \frac{2 \times 5}{3 \times 8} = \frac{10}{24}$$

- Reduce the fraction by dividing the numerator and denominator by the lowest common denominator (2), to find that $X = \frac{5}{12}$.

$$X = \frac{10 \div 2}{24 \div 2} = \frac{5}{12}$$

- Convert $\frac{5}{12}$ to a decimal fraction by dividing the numerator by the denominator, and then rounding it off. The final result is $X = 0.42$.

$$X = \frac{5}{12} = 5 \div 12 = 0.42$$

Add a twist

This example has a twist—the whole number 3 is involved. Here's how to solve for X in the equation:

$$X = \frac{125}{500} \times 3$$

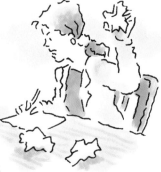

- First, convert the whole number 3 into the fraction $\frac{3}{1}$. (See *Making whole numbers fractions.*) The equation is now:

$$X = \frac{125}{500} \times \frac{3}{1}$$

- Next, reduce $\frac{125}{500}$ by dividing the numerator and denominator by the lowest common denominator (125), to get $\frac{1}{4}$. The equation is now:

$$X = \frac{125 \div 125}{500 \div 125} \times \frac{3}{1}$$

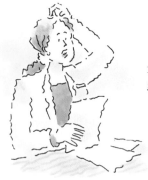

or

$$X = \frac{1}{4} \times \frac{3}{1}$$

- Then proceed as usual. Multiply the numerators:

$$1 \times 3 = 3$$

• Multiply the denominators:

$$4 \times 1 = 4$$

• Restate the equation with this new information:

$$X = \frac{1 \times 3}{4 \times 1} = \frac{3}{4}$$

• The fraction ¾ can't be reduced further. Convert it to a decimal fraction by dividing the numerator by the denominator. The final result is *X* = 0.75.

$$X = \frac{3}{4} = 3 \div 4 = 0.75$$

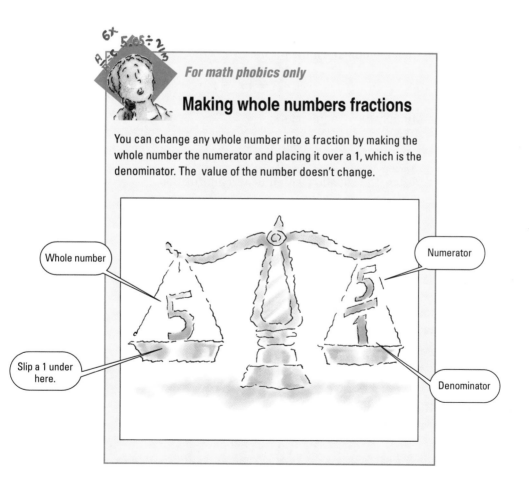

For math phobics only

Making whole numbers fractions

You can change any whole number into a fraction by making the whole number the numerator and placing it over a 1, which is the denominator. The value of the number doesn't change.

Whole number

Numerator

Slip a 1 under here.

Denominator

Solving decimal-fraction equations

To solve for X in equations with decimal fractions, use a method similar to the one above. Here's how to solve for X in the equation:

$$X = \frac{0.05}{0.02} \times 3$$

• First, remove the decimal points from the fraction by moving them two spaces to the right. Then remove the zeros. The equation is now:

$$X = \frac{5}{2} \times 3$$

• Next, convert the whole number 3 to the fraction ³⁄₁. The equation is now:

$$X = \frac{5}{2} \times \frac{3}{1}$$

• Then multiply the numerators:

$$5 \times 3 = 15$$

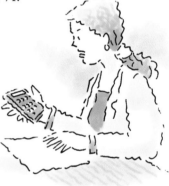

• Multiply the denominators:

$$2 \times 1 = 2$$

• Restate the equation with this new information:

$$X = \frac{5 \times 3}{2 \times 1} = \frac{15}{2}$$

• Convert the answer to decimal form by dividing 15 by 2. The final result is $X = 7.5$.

$$X = \frac{15}{2}$$

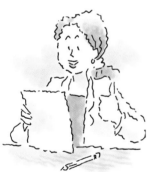

or

$$X = 15 \div 2 = 7.5$$

An X-ample

Here's another practice problem:

$$X = \frac{0.33}{0.11} \times 0.6$$

• Remove the decimal points from the fraction by moving them two spaces to the right. Then remove the zeros. The equation is now:

$$X = \frac{33}{11} \times 0.6$$

• Convert the number 0.6 into the fraction $^{0.6}\!/_1$. The equation is now

$$X = \frac{33}{11} \times \frac{0.6}{1}$$

• Multiply the numerators:

$$33 \times 0.6 = 19.8$$

• Multiply the denominators:

$$11 \times 1 = 11$$

• Restate the equation with this new information:

$$X = \frac{33 \times 0.6}{11 \times 1}$$

or

$$X = \frac{19.8}{11}$$

• Convert the answer to decimal form by dividing 19.8 by 11. The final result is $X = 1.8$.

$$X = 19.8 \div 11 = 1.8$$

Surprise! Another X-ample

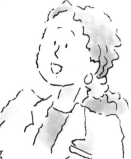

Here's the last problem:

$$X = \frac{0.04}{0.05} \times 4$$

• Remove the decimal points from the fraction by moving them two places to the right. Delete the zeros. The equation is now:

$$X = \frac{4}{5} \times 4$$

• Turn 4 into the fraction $^4\!/_1$. The equation is now:

$$X = \frac{4}{5} \times \frac{4}{1}$$

- Multiply the numerators:

$$4 \times 4 = 16$$

- Multiply the denominators:

$$5 \times 1 = 5$$

- Restate the equation with this new information:

$$X = \frac{4 \times 4}{5 \times 1} = \frac{16}{5}$$

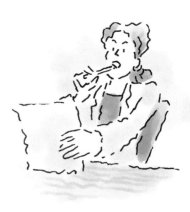

- Convert the answer to decimal form by dividing 16 by 5. The final answer is $X = 3.2$.

$$X = \frac{16}{5}$$

or

$$X = 16 \div 5 = 3.2$$

Solving proportion problems with ratios

A proportion can be written with ratios, as in:

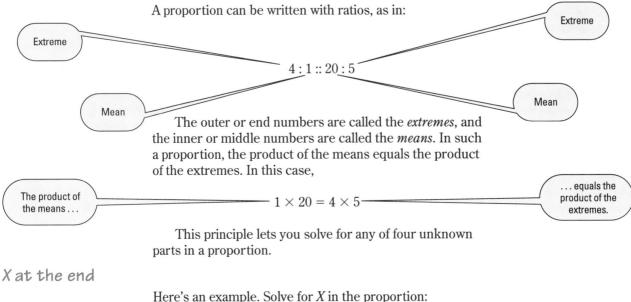

$$4 : 1 :: 20 : 5$$

Extreme

Extreme

Mean

Mean

The outer or end numbers are called the *extremes*, and the inner or middle numbers are called the *means*. In such a proportion, the product of the means equals the product of the extremes. In this case,

The product of the means . . .

$$1 \times 20 = 4 \times 5$$

. . . equals the product of the extremes.

This principle lets you solve for any of four unknown parts in a proportion.

X at the end

Here's an example. Solve for X in the proportion:

$$4 : 8 :: 8 : X$$

Follow these steps:

Rewrite the problem so that the means and the extremes are multiplied:

$$8 \times 8 = 4 \times X$$

Obtain the products of the means and extremes and put them into an equation:

$$64 = 4X$$

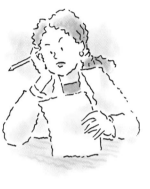

Solve for *X* by dividing both sides by 4. Cancel the number (4) that appears in both the numerator and denominator. This isolates *X* on one side of the equation.

$$\frac{64}{4} = \frac{\cancel{4}X}{\cancel{4}}$$

Find *X*:

$$64 \div 4 = X$$

or

$$X = 16$$

Replace *X* with 16, and restate the proportion in ratios:

$$4 : 8 :: 8 : 16$$

X at the beginning

Solve for *X* in the proportion:

$$X : 12 :: 6 : 24$$

Follow these steps:
• Rewrite the problem so that the means and the extremes are multiplied:

$$12 \times 6 = X \times 24$$

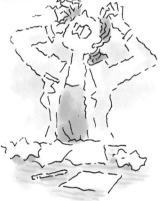

• Obtain the products of the means and extremes, and put them into an equation:

$$72 = 24X$$

• Solve for X by dividing both sides by 24. Cancel the number (24) that appears in both the numerator and denominator. This isolates X on one side of the equation:

$$\frac{72}{24} = \frac{\cancel{24}X}{\cancel{24}}$$

• Find X:

$$72 \div 24 = X$$

or

$$X = 3$$

• Replace X with 24, and restate the proportion in ratios:

$$3 : 12 :: 6 : 24$$

X in the middle

Try one last problem, using this proportion:

$$10 : 20 :: X : 40$$

• Rewrite the problem so that the means and the extremes are multiplied:

$$20 \times X = 10 \times 40$$

• Obtain the products of the means and extremes and put them into an equation:

$$20X = 400$$

• Solve for X by dividing both sides by 20. Cancel the number (20) that appears in both the numerator and denominator. This isolates X on one side of the equation:

$$\frac{\cancel{20}X}{\cancel{20}} = \frac{400}{20}$$

• Find X:

$$X = \frac{400}{20}$$

or

$$X = 20$$

• Replace *X* with 20, and restate the original proportion in ratios:

$$10 : 20 :: 20 : 40$$

Solving proportion problems with fractions

Some people think solving proportion problems is easier with fractions because of their format. In a proportion expressed as a fraction, cross products are equal—just as the means and extremes are equal in a proportion with ratios. (See *Cross product principle*.)

Using the cross products of a proportion, you can solve for any of four unknown parts. Once again, the position of the *X* doesn't matter because the cross products of a proportion are always equal. (See *Cross products to the rescue*, page 60.)

Cross product principle

In a proportion expressed as fractions, cross products are equal. In other words, the numerator on the equation's left side multiplied by the denominator on the equation's right side equals the denominator on the equation's left side multiplied by the numerator on the equation's right side.

The above statement is a lot of words. The same meaning is communicated more simply in the illustration to the left.

Applies to ratios as well

Note that the same principle applies to ratios. In a proportion expressed as ratios, the product of the **means** (numbers in the **middle**) equals the product of the **extremes** (numbers on the **ends**.) Consider the illustration to the right.

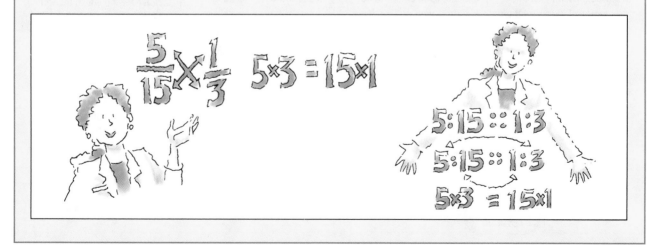

Keeping things in proportion

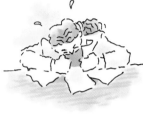

After studying the example in *Cross products to the rescue,* practice solving for X using this proportion:

$$\frac{3}{4} = \frac{9}{X}$$

Follow these steps:
- Rewrite the problem so the cross products are multiplied:

$$3 \times X = 4 \times 9$$

- Obtain the cross products and put them into an equation:

$$3X = 36$$

- Solve for *X* by dividing both sides by 3. Cancel the num-

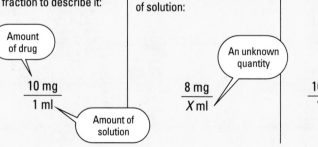

For math phobics only

Cross products to the rescue

Fractions can be used to describe the relative proportion of ingredients, for example the amount of a drug relative to its solution.

Suppose you have a vial containing 10 mg/ml of morphine sulfate. You can write this fraction to describe it:

Amount of drug

$$\frac{10 \text{ mg}}{1 \text{ ml}}$$

Amount of solution

The plot thickens

Now suppose you want to administer 8 mg of morphine sulfate to your patient. How much of the solution should you use?

1. Write a second fraction using *X* to represent the amount of solution:

$$\frac{8 \text{ mg}}{X \text{ ml}}$$

An unknown quantity

2. Set up the equation. Keep the fractions in the same relative proportion of drug to solution.

3. Rewrite the problem so cross products are multiplied:

Cross multiply

$$\frac{10 \text{ mg}}{1 \text{ ml}} \times \frac{8 \text{ mg}}{X \text{ ml}}$$

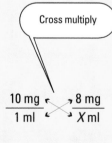

4. This gives you:

$$10X = 8$$

5. Solve for *X* by dividing both sides by 10, and you're left with:

$$X = \frac{8}{10}$$

6. Convert this to a decimal fraction since you'll be drawing up medication and need to work with a decimal:

$$X = 0.8 \text{ ml}$$

The answer

This is how much of the morphine sulfate you should use.

ber (3) that appears in both the numerator and denominator. This isolates X on one side of the equation:

$$\frac{\cancel{3}X}{\cancel{3}} = \frac{36}{3}$$

• Find X:

$$X = \frac{36}{3}$$

or

$$X = 12$$

• Replace the X with 12, and restate the proportion in fractions:

$$\frac{3}{4} = \frac{9}{12}$$

Final practice problem (Yippee!)

Solve one more problem:

$$\frac{12}{25} = \frac{X}{50}$$

• Rewrite the problem so the cross products are multiplied:

$$12 \times 50 = 25 \times X$$

• Obtain the cross products and put them into an equation:

$$600 = 25X$$

• Solve for X by dividing both sides by 25:

$$\frac{600}{25} = \frac{\cancel{25}X}{\cancel{25}}$$

• Find X:

$$X = 24$$

• Replace X with 24, and restate the proportion in fractions:

$$\frac{12}{25} = \frac{24}{50}$$

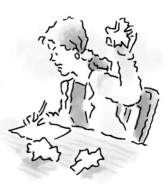

Real world problems

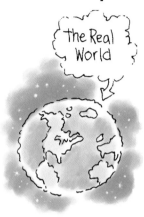

Next, you will find three practical examples of proportions in everyday nursing practice.

How do you set up a proportion to solve a real world problem? Just place the known ratio on one side of the double colon and the unknown ratio on the other side. Be sure that the units of measure in each ratio are in the same positions on both sides of the proportion. (See *Write it down*.)

How much hydrogen peroxide?

Set up a proportion to find out how much hydrogen peroxide (H_2O_2) you should add to 1,000 ml of water (H_2O) to make a solution that contains 50 ml of H_2O_2 for every 100 ml of H_2O.

The ratio approach

To solve this problem using ratios, follow these steps:
• Decide what part of the ratio is X. In this case, it's the amount of H_2O_2 in 1,000 ml of H_2O.
• Set up the proportion so that similar parts of each ratio are in the same position:

$$X \text{ ml } H_2O_2 : 1,000 \text{ ml } H_2O :: 50 \text{ ml } H_2O_2 : 100 \text{ ml } H_2O$$

• Multiply the means and the extremes and restate the problem as an equation:

$$1,000 \text{ ml } H_2O \times 50 \text{ ml } H_2O_2 = X \text{ ml } H_2O_2 \times 100 \text{ ml } H_2O$$

• Solve for X by dividing both sides of the equation by 100 ml H_2O and canceling units that appear in both the numerator and denominator:

$$\frac{1,000 \text{ ml } H_2O \times 50 \text{ ml } H_2O_2}{100 \text{ ml } H_2O} = \frac{X \text{ ml } H_2O_2 \times 100 \text{ ml } H_2O}{100 \text{ ml } H_2O}$$

• Find X:

$$\frac{50,000 \text{ ml } H_2O_2}{100} = X$$

or

$$X = 500 \text{ ml } H_2O_2$$

Write it down

When calculating dosages, you may be able to figure out some problems in your head. For instance, 4 mg in 2 ml is the same as 2 mg in 1 ml. But if you're stumped, don't be shy about writing the proportion down on paper. Taking the time to see the numbers will help you avoid confusion and solve for X more quickly and accurately.

The fraction approach

If you set up a proportion with fractions, place similar units of measure for each fraction in the same position. Here's what the previous example looks like in fraction form:

$$\frac{X \text{ ml } H_2O_2}{1,000 \text{ ml } H_2O} = \frac{50 \text{ ml } H_2O_2}{100 \text{ ml } H_2O}$$

• Rewrite the equation by cross-multiplying the fractions:

$$X \text{ ml } H_2O_2 \times 100 \text{ ml } H_2O = 1,000 \text{ ml } H_2O \times 50 \text{ ml } H_2O_2$$

• Solve for X by dividing both sides of the equation by 100 ml H_2O and canceling units that appear in both the numerator and denominator:

$$\frac{X \text{ ml } H_2O_2 \times \cancel{100 \text{ ml } H_2O}}{\cancel{100 \text{ ml } H_2O}} = \frac{1,000 \cancel{\text{ ml } H_2O} \times 50 \text{ ml } H_2O_2}{100 \cancel{\text{ ml } H_2O}}$$

• Find X:

$$X \text{ ml } H_2O_2 = \frac{50,000 \text{ ml } H_2O_2}{100}$$

$$X = 500 \text{ ml } H_2O_2$$

How many clinical instructors?

Set up another proportion problem with both ratios and fractions. If a school of nursing requires 1 clinical instructor for every 8 students, how many instructors are needed for a class of 24 students?

Resolving it with ratios

Use ratios first. Follow these steps:
• Decide what part of the proportion is X. In this case, it's the number of instructors for 24 students.
• Set up the proportion so that the units of measure (instructors and students) in each ratio are in the same position:

1 instructor : 8 students :: X instructors : 24 students

• Multiply the means and the extremes and set up the equation:

8 students × *X* instructors = 1 instructor × 24 students

• Solve for *X* by dividing both sides of the equation by 8 students and canceling units that appear in both the numerator and denominator:

$$\frac{8 \text{ students} \times X \text{ instructors}}{8 \text{ students}} = \frac{1 \text{ instructor} \times 24 \text{ students}}{8 \text{ students}}$$

• Find *X*:

$$X = 3 \text{ instructors}$$

Figuring it out with fractions

If you prefer to solve the previous problem using fractions, follow these steps:

• Set up the proportion so that the units of measure are in the same position in each fraction. Here's what the problem looks like in fraction form:

$$\frac{1 \text{ instructor}}{8 \text{ students}} = \frac{X \text{ instructors}}{24 \text{ students}}$$

• Rewrite the equation by cross-multiplying the fractions:

1 instructor × 24 students = *X* instructors × 8 students

• Solve for *X* by dividing both sides of the equation by 8 students and canceling units that appear in both the numerator and denominator:

$$\frac{1 \text{ instructor} \times 24 \text{ students}}{8 \text{ students}} = \frac{X \text{ instructors} \times 8 \text{ students}}{8 \text{ students}}$$

$$24 \div 8 = X \text{ instructors}$$

• Find *X*:

$$X = 3 \text{ instructors}$$

How many bags of I.V. fluid?

Here's one more problem. One case of I.V. fluid holds 20 bags. If your home care agency receives 6 cases, how many bags of I.V. fluid does it have?

The ratio rally

Solve this problem using ratios first. Follow these steps:
• Decide what part of the ratio is *X*. In this case, it's the number of bags of I.V. fluid in 6 cases.
• Set up the proportion so that the units of measure in each ratio are in the same position:

$$1 \text{ case} : 20 \text{ bags} :: 6 \text{ cases} : X \text{ bags}$$

• Multiply the means and the extremes and set up the equation:

$$20 \text{ bags} \times 6 \text{ cases} = X \text{ bags} \times 1 \text{ case}$$

• Solve for *X* by dividing both sides of the equation by 1 case and canceling units that appear in both the numerator and denominator:

$$\frac{20 \text{ bags} \times 6 \text{ cases}}{1 \text{ case}} = \frac{X \text{ bags} \times 1 \text{ case}}{1 \text{ case}}$$

$$120 \text{ bags} = X$$

The fraction finale

Now, use fractions to solve the problem. Here's what the equation looks like in fraction form:

$$\frac{1 \text{ case}}{20 \text{ bags}} = \frac{6 \text{ cases}}{X \text{ bags}}$$

• Rewrite the equation by cross-multiplying the fractions. Then solve for *X* by dividing each side of the equation by 1 case and canceling units that appear in both the numerator and denominator:

$$\frac{1 \text{ case} \times X \text{ bags}}{1 \text{ case}} = \frac{6 \text{ cases} \times 20 \text{ bags}}{1 \text{ case}}$$

$$X = 120 \text{ bags}$$

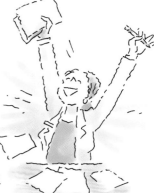

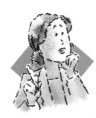

Quick quiz

1. An example of a proportion is:
   A. 4 : 5 :: 8 : 12
   B. 6 : 1 :: 18 : 3
   C. 7 : 1 :: 14 : 7

Answer: B. In a proportion, the ratios equal each other.

2. In fraction form, the proportion 1 : 5 :: 2 : 10 is:
   A. $\frac{1}{5} = \frac{2}{10}$
   B. $\frac{5}{1} = \frac{2}{10}$
   C. $\frac{2}{5} = \frac{1}{10}$

Answer: A. Make the ratios on both sides into fractions by substituting slashes for colons.

3. If a vial has 50 mg of a drug in 5 ml of solution, the amount of drug in 15 ml of solution is:
   A. 10 mg
   B. 150 mg
   C. 75 mg

Answer: B. Substitute *X* for the amount of drug in 15 ml of solution and then set up a proportion with ratios or fractions.

4. The amount of salt you should add to 32 oz of water to make a solution with ½ (0.5) tsp of salt for every 8 oz of water is:
   A. 2 tsp
   B. 4 tsp
   C. 1 tsp

Answer: A. Substitute *X* for the amount of salt in 32 oz of water, and then set up a proportion with ratios or fractions.

Scoring

☆☆☆   If you answered all four items correctly, wow! You're a whiz at relationships (numerical ones, that is).

☆☆   If you answered three or less correctly, all right! You have everything in proportion.

Part II

Measurement systems

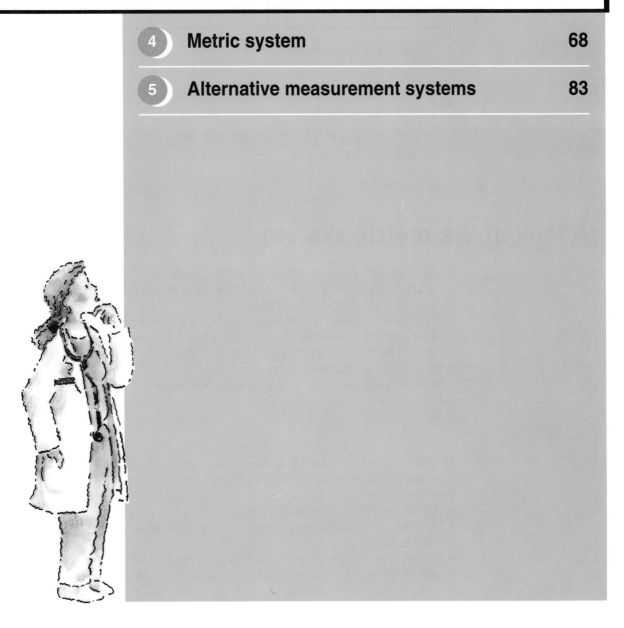

Metric system

Just the facts

In this chapter you'll learn:

♦ the metric units of measure

♦ how to convert measurements from one metric unit to another

♦ how to solve basic arithmetic problems in metric units.

A look at the metric system

Today, most nations of the world rely on the metric system of measurement. It's also the most widely used system for measuring amounts of drugs.

The metric system is a decimal system. That means it's based on the number 10 and multiples of 10. The metric system offers three advantages over other systems:
• It eliminates common fractions.
• It simplifies the calculation of large and small units.
• It simplifies the calculation of drug doses. (See *Tips for going metric*.)

Beginning with the basics

The three basic units of measurement in the metric system (and the abbreviation for each) are the meter (m), the liter (L), and the gram (g).
• The meter is the basic unit of length.
• The liter is the basic unit of volume — it's equivalent to $\frac{1}{10}$ of a cubic meter.
• The gram is the basic unit of weight — it represents the weight of one cubic centimeter of water at 39.2° F (4° C).

What's in a name

All other units of measure are based on these three major units. When you see the root word, *meter, liter,* or *gram* within a measurement, you can easily tell whether you're measuring length, volume, or weight.

For example, the centi*meter* (cm) and the milli*meter* (mm) are units of length, the centi*liter* (cl) and the milli-*liter* (ml) are units of volume, and the kilo*gram* (kg) and the milli*gram* (mg) are units of weight.

Measure for measure

Three devices — the metric ruler, the metric graduate, and metric weights — are used to measure meters, liters, and grams. (See *Measuring meters, liters, and grams,* page 70.)

Building on the basics

The metric system is built on the three basic units: meters, liters, and grams. Multiples and subdivisions of me-

Advice from the experts

Tips for going metric

Remember these tips when using the metric system.

Tip	Example
Use the correct abbreviation for each unit of measurement. The abbreviation always follows a number that represents a quantity.	Five kilograms is abbreviated as 5 kg. Five and one-half milligrams is abbreviated as 5.5 mg.
Use decimal fractions to represent a part of a whole.	2.5 mg represents two milligrams plus five out of ten parts of one milligram.
Place a zero before the decimal point for amounts that are less than 1.	0.5 mg, 0.2 ml, and 0.65 mcg are less than 1.
Eliminate extra zeros so they aren't misread.	Use 5 mg (not 5.0 mg), and 0.5 ml (not 0.500 ml).

ters, liters, and grams are indicated by using a prefix before the basic unit. Each prefix that's used in the metric system represents a multiple or subdivision of ten.

Consider the weighty gram. The most common *multiple* of a gram is the *kilo*gram, which is 1,000 times greater than the gram. The most common *subdivision* of a gram is the *milli*gram, which represents ¹⁄₁,₀₀₀ of a gram or 0.001 gram.

Short, sweet, and marvelously metric

Any metric measurement can be represented by a number and an abbreviation that represents the unit of measure. The abbreviation stands for the basic unit of measure — gram (g), meter (m), liter (L) — and the prefix, such as kilo (k), centi (c), and milli (m). For example, kg stands for kilogram, cm for centimeter, and ml for milliliter. (See *What a little prefix can do*.)

Measuring meters, liters, and grams

What tools do you need to measure meters, liters, and grams? The appropriate measuring devices, of course. A metric ruler, which resembles a yardstick, is used to measure length. A metric graduate can be used to measure the volume of a fluid in liters. (An enclosed chamber, such as a cylinder with a tight-fitting lid, is needed to measure a volume of gas.) A set of metric weights can be used with a metric balance to measure weight in grams.

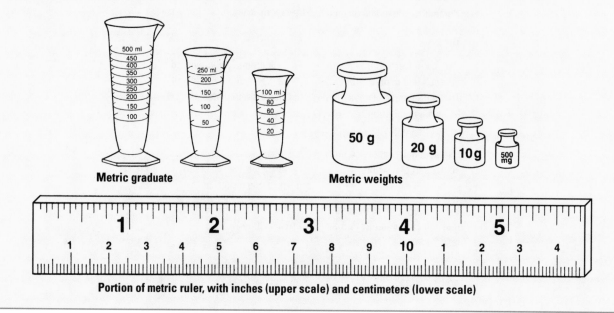

Metric graduate

Metric weights

Portion of metric ruler, with inches (upper scale) and centimeters (lower scale)

One unusual unit

The metric system also includes one unusual unit of volume — the cubic centimeter (cc). Because a cubic centimeter occupies the same space as 1 ml of liquid, the two units of volume are considered equal and may be used interchangeably. However, cubic centimeters usually refer to gas volumes, and milliliters usually describe liquid volumes.

Red alert! Nonstandard abbreviations!

The International Bureau of Weights and Measures adopted the International System of Units in 1960 to promote standard use of metric abbreviations and prevent errors in drug transcriptions. Unfortunately, some health care providers still use the old abbreviations.

So stay alert for nonstandard abbreviations, especially l instead of L to represent liters, and gm or GM instead of g to represent grams. As a precaution, some nurses and doctors use L in all liter-related abbreviations, such as mL and dL. However, this isn't required.

What a little prefix can do

In the metric system, the addition of a prefix to one of the basic units of measure indicates a multiple or subdivision of that unit. Here's a list of prefixes, abbreviations, multiples, and subdivisions of each unit.

Prefix	Abbreviation	Multiples and subdivisions
kilo	k	1,000
hecto	h	100
deka	dk	10
deci	d	0.1 ($\frac{1}{10}$)
centi	c	0.01 ($\frac{1}{100}$)
milli	m	0.001 ($\frac{1}{1,000}$)
micro	mc	0.000001 ($\frac{1}{1,000,000}$)
nano	n	0.000000001 ($\frac{1}{1,000,000,000}$)

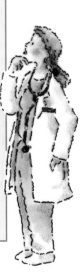

Metric conversions

Because the metric system is decimal based, converting from one metric unit to another is easy. To convert a smaller unit to a larger unit, move the decimal point to the left. To convert a larger unit to a smaller unit, move the decimal point to the right.

Because all metric units are multiples or subdivisions of the major units, you can convert a smaller unit to a larger unit by dividing by the appropriate multiple or multiplying by the appropriate subdivision. To convert a larger unit to a smaller unit, multiply by the appropriate multiple or divide by the appropriate subdivision.

Tour the tables

Luckily, there are tables that you can use to help you to convert measurements. To switch between different units of measure, refer to the *Amazing metric decimal place finder.* You also can speed metric conversions by learning the equivalents of commonly used measures. (See our fabulous *Metric cheat sheet,* page 74.)

Converting meters to kilometers

Suppose you want to convert 15 meters (m) to kilometers (km). Here's how to do it two different ways:

Dancing decimal

Using the *Amazing metric decimal place finder*, follow these steps:
• Count the number of places to the right or left of *meters* to reach *kilo*. You'll see that "kilo" is *three* places to the left, indicating that a kilometer is 1,000 times larger than a meter (note the three zeros in 1,000).
• Move the decimal point in 15.0 three places to the *left,* creating the number 0.015. So, 15 m = 0.015 km. *Remember to place a zero in front of the decimal point to draw attention to the decimal's presence.*

The dividing multiple

Refer to *What a little prefix can do* on page 71. Find "kilo" on the chart. You'll see that it indicates a multiple of 1,000.

Amazing metric decimal place finder

When performing metric conversions, use the following scale as a guide to decimal placement. Each bar represents one decimal place.

When using this chart to go from smaller to larger units (meters to kilometers), you divide by the multiple.

Here's why: One meter multiplied by 1,000 equals 1 kilometer. Think of driving in Europe or Canada; if you drive 1 meter of a 1-kilometer–long road, you're $\frac{1}{1,000}$ of the way there. Therefore, 1 meter equals $\frac{1}{1,000}$ of a kilometer.

To convert 15 meters to kilometers, divide by 1,000. You might want to set up a simple equation:

$$X = \frac{15 \text{ m}}{1,000}$$

$$X = 0.015 \text{ km}$$

So, 15 m = 0.015 km, 15 thousandths of a kilometer.

Converting grams to milligrams

Let's say that you want to convert 5 grams to milligrams. You can use one of two methods.

Decimal dances again

If you use the *Amazing metric decimal place finder* on page 73, follow these steps:
• Count the number of places to the right or left of "grams" to reach "milli." You'll see that "milli" is *three* places to the right, indicating that a milligram is 1,000 times smaller than a gram (note the three zeros in 1,000).
• Move the decimal point in 5.0 three places to the right, creating the number 5,000. So 5 g = 5,000 mg.

The multiplying subdivision

Refer to *What a little prefix can do* on page 71. First, find "milli." You'll see that its subdivision is 0.001, or $\frac{1}{1,000}$. When using this table to go from a larger unit to a smaller unit (such as grams to milligrams), you divide by the subdivision. Here's why: One milligram is $\frac{1}{1,000}$ of a gram. Therefore, 1 gram equals 1,000 milligrams. If you divide 1

Metric cheat sheet

Want a quick way to jump back and forth between different metric measures? Just use the table below. Also, make a copy of it to post in a conspicuous spot on your unit. And always remember, a milliliter is to a liter as a microgram is to a milligram.

Liquids	Solids
1 milliliter = 1 cubic centimeter	1,000 micrograms = 1 milligram
1,000 milliliters = 1 liter	1,000 milligrams = 1 gram
100 centiliters = 1 liter	100 centigrams = 1 gram
10 deciliters = 1 liter	10 decigrams = 1 gram
10 liters = 1 dekaliter	10 grams = 1 dekagram
100 liters = 1 hectoliter	100 grams = 1 hectogram
1,000 liters = 1 kiloliter	1,000 grams = 1 kilogram

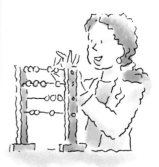

gram by the subdivision ($\frac{1}{1,000}$), you get 1,000 milligrams (dividing by $\frac{1}{1,000}$ is the same as multiplying by 1,000). So to convert 5 g to milligrams, divide 5 g by $\frac{1}{1,000}$ (or multiply it by 1,000).

$$X = \frac{5 \text{ g}}{\frac{1}{1,000}}$$

$$X = 5 \text{ g} \times 1,000$$

$$X = 5,000 \text{ mg}$$

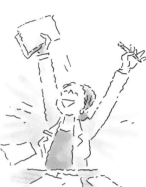

As you can see, 5 g = 5,000 mg.

Converting centiliters to liters

How do you convert 350 cl to liters? Here's how using both charts.

Dancing decimal never rests

Using the *Amazing metric decimal place finder* on page 73, follow these steps:
• Count the number of places to the right or left of "centi" to reach "liters." You'll see that "liters" is two places to the left, indicating that a liter is 100 times larger than a centiliter.
• To show this, move the decimal point in 350.0 two places to the left, creating the number 3.5. So, 350 cl = 3.5 L.

Subdivision multiplies again

Now refer to *What a little prefix can do* on page 71. First, find "centi." You'll see that its subdivision is 0.01 or $\frac{1}{100}$. When using this chart to go from a smaller unit to a larger one (centiliters to liters), you multiply by the subdivision.
Here's why: One liter equals 100 centiliters. Therefore, 1 centiliter is 1/100th of a liter (or 1 liter divided by 100). To convert 350 centiliters to liters, multiply 350 cl by $\frac{1}{100}$ (which is the same as dividing by 100) to get 3.5 L.

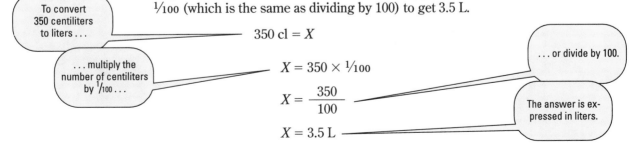

To convert 350 centiliters to liters . . .

. . . multiply the number of centiliters by $\frac{1}{100}$ . . .

$$350 \text{ cl} = X$$

$$X = 350 \times \frac{1}{100}$$

$$X = \frac{350}{100}$$

$$X = 3.5 \text{ L}$$

. . . or divide by 100.

The answer is expressed in liters.

Solving for *X*

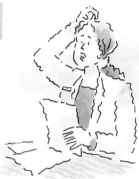

Another way to convert between metric units is by solving for *X*. The following examples show how to solve for *X* in three clinical situations.

How much does that baby weigh?

An infant weighs 6.5 kg. How much does he weigh in grams? To solve the problem, follow these steps:
• First, refer to the *Metric cheat sheet* on page 74. You'll see that 1,000 g equals 1 kg.
• Now set up the following equation, substituting *X* for the unknown weight in grams.

$$\frac{1{,}000 \text{ g}}{1 \text{ kg}} = \frac{X \text{ g}}{6.5 \text{ kg}}$$

• Cross-multiply the fractions

$$\frac{1{,}000 \text{ g}}{1 \text{ kg}} \diagup\!\!\!\!\diagdown \frac{X \text{ g}}{6.5 \text{ kg}}$$

$$X \text{ g} \times 1 \text{ kg} = 6.5 \text{ kg} \times 1{,}000 \text{ g}$$

• Divide both sides of the equation by 1 kg, to isolate *X*. Cancel units that appear in both the numerator and denominator:

$$\frac{X \text{ g} \times \cancel{1 \text{ kg}}}{\cancel{1 \text{ kg}}} = \frac{6.5 \cancel{\text{ kg}} \times 1{,}000 \text{ g}}{1 \cancel{\text{ kg}}}$$

$$X = 6{,}500 \text{ g}$$

The infant weighs 6,500 g.

How much I.V. fluid?

If a patient received 0.375 L of lactated Ringer's solution, how many milliliters did he receive?
• Refer to the *Metric cheat sheet* on page 74. You'll see that 1 L is equal to 1,000 ml.
• Now set up the following equation, substituting *X* for the unknown amount of I.V. solution in milliliters:

$$\frac{1 \text{ L}}{1{,}000 \text{ ml}} = \frac{0.375 \text{ L}}{X \text{ ml}}$$

• Cross-multiply the fractions:

$$\frac{1\,\text{L}}{1{,}000\,\text{ml}} \;\diagdown\!\!\!\!\diagup\; \frac{0.375\,\text{L}}{X\,\text{ml}}$$

$$X\,\text{ml} \times 1\,\text{L} = 0.375\,\text{L} \times 1{,}000\,\text{ml}$$

• Divide both sides of the equation by 1 L, to isolate *X*. Cancel units that appear in both the numerator and denominator:

$$\frac{X\,\text{ml} \times \cancel{1\,\text{L}}}{\cancel{1\,\text{L}}} = \frac{0.375\,\cancel{\text{L}} \times 1{,}000\,\text{ml}}{1\,\cancel{\text{L}}}$$

$$X = 375\,\text{ml}$$

• The patient received 375 ml of I.V. fluid.

How much medication?

A nurse administered 2 g of ceftriaxone sodium (Rocephin). How many milligrams of this medication did the patient receive?
• Refer to the *Metric cheat sheet* on page 74. You'll see that 1 g is equal to 1,000 mg.
• Now set up the following equation, substituting *X* for the unknown amount of medication in milligrams:

$$\frac{1\,\text{g}}{1{,}000\,\text{mg}} = \frac{2\,\text{g}}{X\,\text{mg}}$$

• Cross-multiply the fractions:

$$\frac{1\,\text{g}}{1{,}000\,\text{mg}} \;\diagdown\!\!\!\!\diagup\; \frac{2\,\text{g}}{X\,\text{mg}}$$

$$X\,\text{mg} \times 1\,\text{g} = 2\,\text{g} \times 1{,}000\,\text{mg}$$

• Divide each side of the equation by 1 g, to isolate *X*. Cancel units that appear in both the numerator and denominator:

$$\frac{X\,\text{mg} \times \cancel{1\,\text{g}}}{\cancel{1\,\text{g}}} = \frac{2\,\cancel{\text{g}} \times 1{,}000\,\text{mg}}{1\,\cancel{\text{g}}}$$

$$X = 2{,}000\,\text{mg}$$

The patient received 2,000 mg of Rocephin.

Metric mathematics

To add, subtract, multiply, or divide different metric units, first convert all quantities to the same unit. Unless the problem calls for an answer in a specific unit, use the common unit that's easiest for you to work with, and then perform the arithmetic.

For example, suppose you want to add 2 kg, 202 mg, and 222 g, expressing the total in grams. Here's how to do this:
• First convert all the measurements to grams. Refer to the *Metric cheat sheet* on page 74.
• 1 kg equals 1,000 g. Therefore, you can multiply 2 kg by 1,000 to get 2,000 g.
• 1,000 mg equals 1 g and 1 mg equals $1/1,000$ g. Therefore, you can divide 202 mg by 1,000 to get 0.202 g.
• Now do the addition:

$$2,000 + 0.202 + 222 = 2,222.202 \text{ g}$$

Real world problems

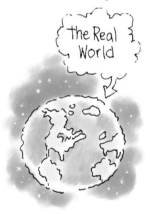

the Real World

A patient with a liter bag of I.V. fluid received 500 ml of fluid over the first shift, 225 ml over the second shift, and 150 ml over the third shift. How many milliliters of fluid remain in the I.V. bag?
• First determine how much fluid the patient received. To do this, add:

$$500 + 225 + 150 = 875 \text{ ml}$$

• Because you're trying to determine the number of milliliters remaining, you need only convert 1 L to milliliters. Refer to the *Metric cheat sheet* on page 74, where you'll see that 1 L = 1,000 ml.
• Finally, compute the amount of fluid remaining in the I.V. bag by subtracting 875 ml from 1,000 ml. The answer is 125 ml.

Example extraordinaire: A tantalizing tablet tabulation!

A patient is to receive 5 g of erythromycin (Erythrocin) before intestinal surgery. If erythromycin is available in 500-mg tablets, how many tablets should be administered?

• First, convert all the measures to the same units. Because you're trying to determine the number of 500-mg tablets to administer, convert 5 g to milligrams. Refer to the *Metric cheat sheet* on page 74 where you'll see that 1 g is equal to 1,000 mg.

• To find how many milligrams are in 5 g, set up this proportion using fractions:

$$\frac{1,000 \text{ mg}}{1 \text{ g}} = \frac{X \text{ mg}}{5 \text{ g}}$$

• Then cross-multiply the fractions and divide each side of the resulting equation by 1 g to solve for X. You find that X is 5,000 mg:

$$\frac{1,000 \text{ mg}}{1 \text{ g}} \diagup\!\!\!\!\diagdown \frac{X \text{ mg}}{5 \text{ g}}$$

$$X \text{ mg} \times 1 \text{ g} = 1,000 \text{ mg} \times 5 \text{ g}$$

$$\frac{X \text{ mg} \times 1\text{g}}{1\text{g}} = \frac{1,000 \text{ mg} \times 5\text{g}}{1\text{g}}$$

$$X = 5,000 \text{ mg}$$

• To determine the number of 500-mg tablets that need to be administered to provide 5,000 mg, set up another proportion using fractions:

$$\frac{500 \text{ mg}}{1 \text{ tablet}} = \frac{5,000 \text{ mg}}{X \text{ tablets}}$$

• Cross-multiply the fractions and divide each side of the resulting equation by 500 mg to solve for X. You find that X is 10 tablets:

$$\frac{500 \text{ mg}}{1 \text{ tablet}} \diagup\!\!\!\!\diagdown \frac{5,000 \text{ mg}}{X \text{ tablets}}$$

$$500 \text{ mg} \times X \text{ tablets} = 5,000 \text{ mg} \times 1 \text{ tablet}$$

$$\frac{X \text{ tablets} \times 500 \text{ mg}}{500 \text{ mg}} = \frac{1 \text{ tablet} \times 5,000 \text{ mg}}{500 \text{ mg}}$$

$$X = 10 \text{ tablets}$$

You should administer 10 tablets of erythromycin.

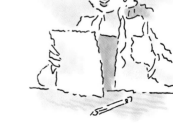

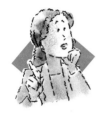

Quick quiz

1. Gram, meter, and liter respectively measure:
    A. length, volume, and weight.
    B. weight, length, and volume.
    C. volume, weight, and length.

Answer: B. Gram, meter, and liter — the three basic units of the metric system — measure weight, length, and volume respectively.

2. An order written according to the International System of Units would read:
    A. gentamicin 400 mg in 100 ML normal saline I.V. q 24 hours.
    B. gentamicin (Gentacidin) 400 mG in 100 mL normal saline I.V. q 24 hours.
    C. gentamicin 400 mg in 100 ml normal saline I.V. q 24 hours.

Answer: C. According to the International System of Units, mg and ml are the standard metric abbreviations.

3. To convert milligrams to grams, move the decimal point:
    A. three places to the left.
    B. three places to the right.
    C. two places to the left.

Answer: A. Locate milli- and grams on the *Amazing metric decimal place finder* on page 73, count the number of places grams is to the left of milli-, and then move the decimal point accordingly.

4. The number of milligrams in 3,120 mcg is:
    A. 3,120,000 mg
    B. 0.312 mg
    C. 3.12 mg

Answer: C. Locate milli- and micro- on the *Amazing metric decimal place finder* on page 73, count the number of places milli- is to the left of micro-, and then move the decimal point three places to the left.

5. The total volume in milliliters of 312 ml, 3.12 L, and 312 L is:
    A. 327.12 ml

B. 315,432 ml

C. 31,543.2 L

Answer: B. Convert all the measures to milliliters, and then add all three numbers.

6. The measure that's equivalent to a milliliter is:
   A. a cubic centimeter.
   B. a kiloliter.
   C. a hectoliter.

Answer: A. A milliliter of liquid occupies a cubic centimeter of space.

7. The weight in grams of a baby that weighs 5.2 kg is:
   A. 5.2 g
   B. 5.02 g
   C. 5,200 g

Answer: C. Knowing that 1 kg is equal to 1,000 g, set up an equation with X g as the unknown quantity, and multiply 5.2 kg by 1,000 g/kg.

8. The number of milliters left in a 4-liter bag of normal saline solution after you remove 50 ml, 250 ml, 2.5 L, and 750 ml is:
   A. 3,550 ml
   B. 450 ml
   C. 50 ml

Answer: B. Convert all the measurements to milliliters, add the last four numbers to find out how many milliters were removed from the bag, and then subtract this number from the amount of fluid in the bag.

9. The smallest metric measurement is the:
   A. micro.
   B. deci.
   C. nano.

Answer: C. The nano measures billionths.

10. The number of milligrams of imipenem (Primaxin) remaining in a 5-g vial after 250 mg are removed is:
    A. 4,750 mg
    B. 47 mg
    C. 4 g

Answer: A. Convert all the measurements to milligrams, and set up an equation with X mg as the unknown quantity. Multiply 5 g by 1,000 mg to get 5,000 mg, and then subtract 250 from 5,000 to get the amount left in the vial.

Scoring

☆☆☆ If you answered all 10 items correctly, give yourself 10 points! If each point were equal to a gram, you'd have 10 grams, or 100 decigrams, or 1,000 centigrams, or 10,000 milligrams, or 10,000,000 micrograms.

☆☆ If you answered seven to nine correctly, dig those decimals! You are a metric master!

☆ If you answered fewer than seven correctly, leapin' milliliters! You'll soon be doing a hecto of a good job!

Alternative measurement systems

Just the facts

In this chapter, you'll learn:

♦ what the apothecaries' system is and how it works

♦ what the household system is and how it works

♦ what the avoirdupois system is and how it works

♦ what the unit system is and how it works

♦ what the milliequivalent system is and how it works

♦ how to perform common conversions.

A look at alternative systems

Although the metric system is used most often in clinical settings, you'll work with other systems from time to time. These systems include the apothecaries', household, avoirdupois, unit, and milliequivalent systems.

When the alternative is the answer

When would you use these other systems? For example, you might:
• receive a drug order written using the apothecaries' system
• teach a patient to use a measuring device calibrated in the household system
• use the avoirdupois system to calculate a dose that's based on a patient's weight.

You can prepare yourself for these occasions by familiarizing yourself with alternative measurement systems.

Apothecaries' system

Doctors and pharmacists used the apothecaries' system before the metric system was introduced. Since then, use of the older system has declined. But even though this system is rarely seen anymore, you should still be familiar with it.

Basic minims and grains

Unlike the metric system, which is used to measure length, volume, and weight, the apothecaries' system is used to measure only liquid volumes and solid weights. The basic unit for measuring liquid volume is the minim, and the basic unit for measuring solid weight is the grain.

A drop in the grain bucket

One way to remember these units is to visualize the minim as about the size of a drop of water, which weighs about the same as a grain of wheat. The following mathematical statement sums up this relationship:

$$1 \text{ drop} = 1 \text{ minim} = 1 \text{ grain}$$

Other units of measure in the apothecaries' system build on these two basic units. Many of these units are also common household measures. (See *Ye olde apothecaries' system.*)

Dram it: Apothecaries' conversions

Measurements of liquids and solids that are expressed in the apothecaries' system can easily be converted from one unit of measure to another. Here are a few examples:
1. *How many fluid drams are in 60 minims?* From the table shown in *Ye olde apothecaries' system,* you can see that 60 minims equal 1 fluid dram.
2. *How many quarts are in 1 gallon?* One gallon equals 4 quarts of fluid.
3. *How many drams are in 30 grains?* Because 60 grains equal 1 dram, 30 grains equal ½ dram.

I prefer to use Ye Olde Calculator!

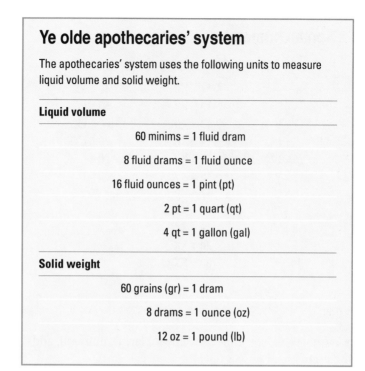

Ye olde apothecaries' system

The apothecaries' system uses the following units to measure liquid volume and solid weight.

Liquid volume

60 minims = 1 fluid dram

8 fluid drams = 1 fluid ounce

16 fluid ounces = 1 pint (pt)

2 pt = 1 quart (qt)

4 qt = 1 gallon (gal)

Solid weight

60 grains (gr) = 1 dram

8 drams = 1 ounce (oz)

12 oz = 1 pound (lb)

Roman numerals

Some doctors and pharmacists express apothecaries' system dosages in Arabic numerals followed by units of measure. However, the apothecaries' system traditionally uses Roman numerals. (See *Roman numerals*, page 86.)

When in Rome...

When used in pharmacologic applications, Roman numerals ss through x usually are written in lower case. When Roman numerals are used, the unit of measure goes before the numeral. For example, 5 grains is written grains v. Fractions of less than ½ are written as common fractions using Arabic numerals. Other quantities are expressed by combining letters according to two general rules:
• When a smaller numeral precedes a larger numeral, subtract the smaller numeral from the larger numeral. For example:

$$IX = 10 - 1 = 9$$

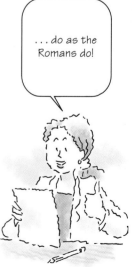

...do as the Romans do!

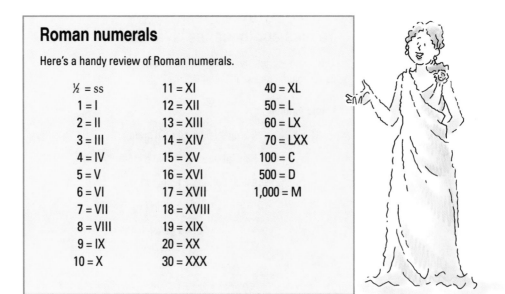

Roman numerals

Here's a handy review of Roman numerals.

½ = ss	11 = XI	40 = XL
1 = I	12 = XII	50 = L
2 = II	13 = XIII	60 = LX
3 = III	14 = XIV	70 = LXX
4 = IV	15 = XV	100 = C
5 = V	16 = XVI	500 = D
6 = VI	17 = XVII	1,000 = M
7 = VII	18 = XVIII	
8 = VIII	19 = XIX	
9 = IX	20 = XX	
10 = X	30 = XXX	

• When a smaller numeral follows a larger numeral, add the numerals. For example:

$$XI = 10 + 1 = 11$$

Breaking up is easy to do

To convert an Arabic numeral to a Roman numeral, first break the Arabic numeral into its component parts; then translate each part into Roman numerals. For example:

$$36 = 30 + 6 = XXX + VI = XXXVI$$

Roman numeral conversions

Now that you understand how Roman numerals work, convert the numbers below:

1. *Write 53 using Roman numerals:*

$$53 = 50 + 3 = L + III = LIII$$

2. *Write CXXVI using Arabic numerals:*

$$CXXVI = C + X + X + VI = 100 + 10 + 10 + 6 = 126$$

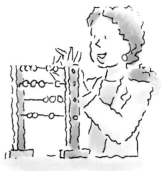

3. *Write 1,558 using Roman numerals:*

$$1{,}558 = 1{,}000 + 500 + 50 + 8 = M + D + L + VIII = MDLVIII$$

Household system

The household system of measurement uses droppers, teaspoons, tablespoons, and cups to measure liquid medication doses. (See *Making sure the cup doesn't runneth over,* page 88.) However, because these measuring devices aren't all alike, the household system is useful only for approximate measurements. For exact measurements, use the metric system.

To measure drug doses at home, the patient uses the household system. So teach him to measure the prescribed dose using household measures. (See *A spoonful of sugar,* page 89.)

Household system conversions

The examples below show how to convert measurements using the household system.

Cough syrup conundrum

The doctor has ordered *120 drops (gtt) of an expectorant cough syrup every 6 hours* for your patient. The drug label gives instructions in teaspoons. How many teaspoons should you administer?

• There are 60 gtt of liquid in 1 teaspoon (tsp). To find out how many teaspoons are in 120 gtt, set up the following equation, using X as the unknown quantity:

$$\frac{60 \text{ gtt}}{1 \text{ tsp}} = \frac{120 \text{ gtt}}{X \text{ tsp}}$$

• Cross-multiply the fractions:

$$X \text{ tsp} \times 60 \text{ gtt} = 1 \text{ tsp} \times 120 \text{ gtt}$$

• Solve for X by dividing both sides of the equation by

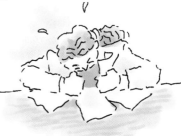

60 gtt and canceling units that appear in both the numerator and denominator:

$$\frac{X \text{ tsp} \times 60\,\cancel{\text{gtt}}}{60\,\cancel{\text{gtt}}} = \frac{1 \text{ tsp} \times 120\,\cancel{\text{gtt}}}{60\,\cancel{\text{gtt}}}$$

$$X = \frac{1 \text{ tsp} \times 120}{60}$$

$$X = 2 \text{ tsp}$$

The patient should receive 2 tsp of cough syrup.

Broth brain teaser

Your patient is on a clear diet. For lunch he drank 6 tablespoons (tbs) of chicken broth. How many ounces did he consume?

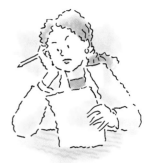

▶ *Teaching points*

Making sure the cup doesn't runneth over

Will your patient be taking medication at home? If so, teach him to use the devices below to help ensure accurate measurements.

Medication cup
A medication cup is calibrated in household, metric, and apothecaries' systems. Tell the patient to set the cup on a counter or flat surface and to check the fluid measurement at eye level.

Dropper
A dropper is calibrated in household or metric systems or in terms of medication strength or concentration. Advise the patient to hold the dropper at eye level to check the fluid measurement.

Hollow-handle spoon
A hollow-handle spoon is calibrated in teaspoons and tablespoons. Teach the patient to check the dose after filling by holding the spoon upright at eye level. Instruct him to administer the medication by tilting the spoon until the medicine fills the bowl of the spoon and then placing the spoon in his mouth.

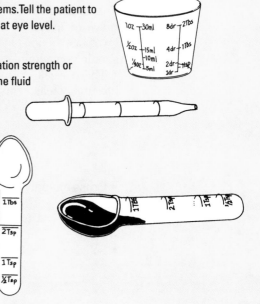

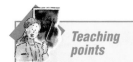

• There are 2 tbs of liquid in 1 ounce (oz). To find out how many ounces are in 6 tbs, set up the following equation, using *X* as the unknown quantity:

$$\frac{2\text{ tbs}}{1\text{ oz}} = \frac{6\text{ tbs}}{X\text{ oz}}$$

• Cross-multiply the fractions:

$$X\text{ oz} \times 2\text{ tbs} = 1\text{ oz} \times 6\text{ tbs}$$

• Find *X* by dividing each side of the equation by 2 tbs and canceling units that appear in both the numerator and denominator:

$$\frac{X\text{ oz} \times 2\text{ tbs}}{2\text{ tbs}} = \frac{1\text{ oz} \times 6\text{ tbs}}{2\text{ tbs}}$$

$$X = 3\text{ oz}$$

The patient consumed 3 oz of chicken broth.

Milk of magnesia mystery

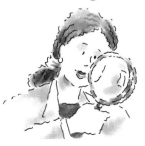

Your patient is to receive 4 tbs of milk of magnesia. This is equal to how many teaspoons?
• There are 3 tsp of liquid in 1 tbs. To find out how many teaspoons are in 4 tbs, set up the following equation using *X* as the unknown quantity:

$$\frac{3\text{ tsp}}{1\text{ tbs}} = \frac{X\text{ tsp}}{4\text{ tbs}}$$

• Solve for *X* by cross-multiplying the fractions, then dividing each side of the equation by 1 tbs, and canceling units that appear in both the numerator and denominator:

$$\frac{X\text{ tsp} \times 1\text{ tbs}}{1\text{ tbs}} = \frac{3\text{ tsp} \times 4\text{ tbs}}{1\text{ tbs}}$$

$$X = 12\text{ tsp}$$

The patient gets 12 tsp of milk of magnesia.

Avoirdupois system

This difficult-to-pronounce system of measurement (av-wah-doo-PWAH) is used for ordering and purchasing some pharmaceutical products and for weighing patients.

In this system, the solid measures or units of weight include grains, ounces, and pounds. One ounce equals 480 grains, and 1 lb equals 16 oz or 7,680 grains. Note that the apothecaries' pound equals 12 oz, but the avoirdupois pound equals 16 oz. (See *Measure for measure.*)

Avoirdupois system conversions

The following examples show how to perform conversions in the avoirdupois system:

1. *How many pounds equal 32 oz?* One pound equals 16 oz; therefore, 2 lb equal 32 oz.

2. *How many ounces equal 7,680 grains?* One pound equals 7,680 grains; therefore, 16 oz equal 7,680 grains.

3. *How many grains are in 2 lb?* You know that 7,680 grains are in 1 lb; therefore, 15,360 grains are in 2 lb.

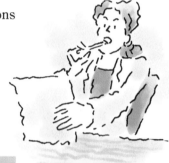

Unit system

Some drugs are measured in units (U), such as United States Pharmacopeia (USP) units or International Units (IU). The most common drug that's measured in units is insulin, which comes in 10-ml multidose vials of U-40 or U-100 strength.

With insulin, the U refers to the number of units per milliliter. For example, 1 ml of U-40 insulin contains 40 units, and 1 ml of U-100 insulin contains 100 units. Use of U-40 insulin has declined in recent years; the U-100 strength, which is based on metric measurements, makes measurement in a standard syringe easier.

Some other drugs are also measured in units; for example, the anticoagulant heparin, the topical antibiotic bacitracin, and penicillin G and V. The hormone calcitonin and the fat-soluble vitamins A, D, and E are measured in IU. Some forms of vitamin A and D are also measured in USP units.

Measure for measure

Here are some approximate liquid and solid equivalents among the household, apothecaries', avoirdupois, and metric systems. Use your facility's protocol for converting measurements from one system to another.

Liquids

Household	Apothecaries'	Metric
1 drop (gtt)	1 minim (m)	0.06 millimeter (ml)
15 to 16 gtt	15 to 16 m	1 ml
1 teaspoon (tsp)	1 fluid dram	4 or 5 ml
1 tablespoon (tbs)	½ fluid ounce	15 or 16 ml
2 tbs	1 fluid ounce	30 or 32 ml
1 cup	8 fluid ounces	240 or 250 ml
1 pint (pt)	16 fluid ounces	473, 480, or 500 ml
1 quart (qt)	32 fluid ounces	946, 960, or 1,000 ml (1 liter)
1 gallon (gal)	128 fluid ounces	3,785, 3,840, or 4,000 ml

Solids

Avoirdupois	Apothecaries'	Metric
1 grain (gr)	1 grain	0.06 or 0.065 gram (g)
15.4 grains	15 grains	1 g
1 oz	480 grains	28.35 g
1 pound (lb)	1.33 lb	454 g
2.2 lb	2.7 lb	1 kilogram

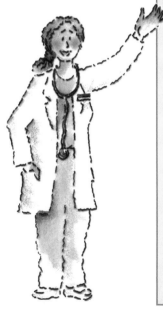

All out of proportion

To calculate the dose to be administered when the medication is available in units, use the following proportion:

$$\frac{\text{amount of drug in ml or other measure}}{\text{dose required in U}} = \frac{\text{1 ml or other measure}}{\text{drug available in U}}$$

Unit system conversions

The examples below show how to perform conversions in the unit system.

Drip...drip...drip...

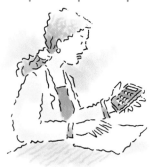

A standard heparin drip of 25,000 U in 500 ml of half normal saline solution is ordered for your patient. The heparin vial that's available has 5,000 U/ml. How many milliliters of heparin should you add to the I.V. fluid? Here's how to solve this problem:

• Set up a proportion using X as the unknown quantity:

$$\frac{X \text{ ml}}{25,000 \text{ U}} = \frac{1 \text{ ml}}{5,000 \text{ U}}$$

• Cross-multiply the fractions:

$$X \text{ ml} \times 5,000 \text{ U} = 1 \text{ ml} \times 25,000 \text{ U}$$

• Find X by dividing both sides of the equation by 5,000 U and canceling units that appear in both the numerator and denominator:

$$\frac{X \text{ ml} \times \cancel{5,000 \text{ U}}}{\cancel{5,000 \text{ U}}} = \frac{1 \text{ ml} \times 25,000 \cancel{\text{U}}}{5,000 \cancel{\text{U}}}$$

$$X = 5 \text{ ml}$$

You should add 5 ml of heparin to the I.V. fluid.

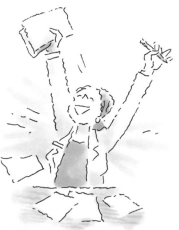

Penicillin problem

Your patient needs 500,000 U of penicillin by deep intra-muscular injection. The vial of penicillin that's available contains 1,000,000 U/ml. How much of the drug should you draw up? Here's how to solve this problem:
• Set up a proportion using X as the unknown quantity:

$$\frac{X \text{ ml}}{500,000 \text{ U}} = \frac{1 \text{ ml}}{1,000,000 \text{ U}}$$

• Cross-multiply the fractions:

$$X \text{ ml} \times 1,000,000 \text{ U} = 1 \text{ ml} \times 500,000 \text{ U}$$

• Find X by dividing each side of the equation by 1,000,000 U and canceling units that appear in both the numerator and denominator:

$$\frac{X \text{ ml} \times \cancel{1,000,000 \text{ U}}}{\cancel{1,000,000 \text{ U}}} = \frac{1 \text{ ml} \times 500,000 \cancel{\text{ U}}}{1,000,000 \cancel{\text{ U}}}$$

$$X = 0.5 \text{ ml}$$

You need to inject 0.5 ml of penicillin.

Milliliter mystery

The doctor orders *a bolus of 3,000 U of heparin* for your patient. The heparin vial that's available contains 1,000 U/ml. How many milliliters should you administer?
• Set up a proportion using X as the unknown quantity of heparin:

$$\frac{X \text{ ml}}{3,000 \text{ U}} = \frac{1 \text{ ml}}{1,000 \text{ U}}$$

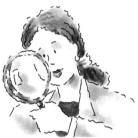

• Cross-multiply the fractions:

$$X \text{ ml} \times 1,000 \text{ U} = 1 \text{ ml} \times 3,000 \text{ U}$$

• Find X by dividing both sides of the equation by 1,000 U and canceling units that appear in both the numerator and denominator:

$$\frac{X \text{ ml} \times \cancel{1,000 \text{ U}}}{\cancel{1,000 \text{ U}}} = \frac{1 \text{ ml} \times 3,000 \cancel{\text{ U}}}{1,000 \cancel{\text{ U}}}$$

$$X = 3 \text{ ml}$$

You should administer a 3-ml bolus of heparin.

Milliequivalent system

Electrolytes are measured in milliequivalents (mEq). Drug manufacturers dispense information about the number of metric units required to provide the prescribed number of milliequivalents. For example, the manufacturer's instructions may indicate that 1 ml equals 4 mEq.

A doctor usually orders the electrolyte potassium chloride in milliequivalents. Potassium preparations are available for use in I.V. fluids, as oral suspensions or elixirs, and in solid tablets or powder form. Potassium is also available in the combination drug potassium phosphorus. The phosphorus in this drug is measured in millimoles.

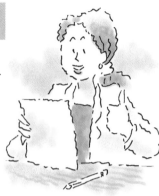

A propitious proportion

To calculate the dose to be administered when the medication is available in milliequivalents, use the proportion:

$$\frac{\text{amount of drug in ml or other measure}}{\text{dose required in mEq}} = \frac{\text{1 ml or other measure}}{\text{drug available in mEq}}$$

Milliequivalent system conversions

The problems below show how to do conversions using the milliequivalent system.

Salty solution

The doctor has ordered an *I.V. infusion of 40 mEq of potassium chloride in 100 ml of normal saline solution* for your patient. The potassium vial that's available contains 10 mEq/ml. How many milliliters of potassium chloride should you infuse? Here's how to solve this problem:
• Set up a proportion using X as the unknown quantity:

$$\frac{X \text{ ml}}{40 \text{ mEq}} = \frac{1 \text{ ml}}{10 \text{ mEq}}$$

• Cross-multiply the fractions:

$$X \text{ ml} \times 10 \text{ mEq} = 1 \text{ ml} \times 40 \text{ mEq}$$

- Find X by dividing each side of the equation by 10 mEq and canceling units that appear in both the numerator and denominator:

$$\frac{X \text{ ml} \times 10 \text{ mEq}}{10 \text{ mEq}} = \frac{1 \text{ ml} \times 40 \text{ mEq}}{10 \text{ mEq}}$$

$$X = 4 \text{ ml}$$

You need to dilute 4 ml of potassium chloride in the normal saline solution.

Break for baking soda

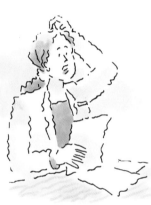

Your patient needs 25 mEq of sodium bicarbonate. The vial from the pharmacy contains 50 mEq in every 50 ml. How many milliliters of the solution should you administer? Here's how to solve this problem:
- Set up a proportion using X as the unknown quantity:

$$\frac{X \text{ ml}}{25 \text{ mEq}} = \frac{50 \text{ ml}}{50 \text{ mEq}}$$

- Cross-multiply the fractions:

$$X \text{ ml} \times 50 \text{ mEq} = 50 \text{ ml} \times 25 \text{ mEq}$$

- Find X by dividing both sides of the equation by 50 mEq and canceling units that appear in both the numerator and denominator:

$$\frac{X \text{ ml} \times 50 \text{ mEq}}{50 \text{ mEq}} = \frac{50 \text{ ml} \times 25 \text{ mEq}}{50 \text{ mEq}}$$

$$X = 25 \text{ ml}$$

You should administer 25 ml of sodium bicarbonate.

Potassium puzzle

The doctor prescribes *30 mEq of potassium chloride oral solution* for your patient. The solution contains 60 mEq in every 15 ml. How many milliliters of solution should you give the patient? Here's how to solve this problem:
- Set up a proportion using X as the unknown quantity:

$$\frac{X \text{ ml}}{30 \text{ mEq}} = \frac{15 \text{ ml}}{60 \text{ mEq}}$$

• Cross-multiply the fractions:

$$X \text{ ml} \times 60 \text{ mEq} = 15 \text{ ml} \times 30 \text{ mEq}$$

• Find X by dividing both sides of the equation by 60 mEq and canceling units that appear in both the numerator and denominator:

$$\frac{X \text{ ml} \times \cancel{60 \text{ mEq}}}{\cancel{60 \text{ mEq}}} = \frac{15 \text{ ml} \times 30 \cancel{\text{ mEq}}}{60 \cancel{\text{ mEq}}}$$

$$X = 7.5 \text{ ml}$$

You should administer 7.5 ml of oral potassium chloride.

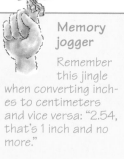

Memory jogger

Remember this jingle when converting inches to centimeters and vice versa: "2.54, that's 1 inch and no more."

Frequently used conversions

In clinical practice, a doctor may write a medication order in one measurement system, but the medication may be available in a different system. For example, he might order 10 grains of a drug that's available only in milligrams.

To convert medication orders from one system to another, you must know the equivalent measures. If you have trouble remembering the most frequently used equivalents, jot the equivalents on an index card, laminate the card, and tuck it into your pocket along with your calculator for easy reference.

A conversion excursion

Two conversions that are frequently used, especially in adult and pediatric intensive care units, are pounds (lb) to kilograms (kg) and inches to centimeters (cm). These conversions are used to determine body weight and body surface, not to calculate dosage.

Making these conversions isn't hard if you remember these general rules:
• Remember that 1 kg equals 2.2 lb. To convert pounds into kilograms, just divide the number of pounds by 2.2.
• To convert kilograms to pounds, multiply the number of kilograms by 2.2.
• Remember that 1″ equals 2.54 cm. To convert inches to centimeters, just multiply the number of inches by 2.54 cm.

• To convert centimeters to inches, divide the number of centimeters by 2.54.

Equivalent measure conversions

The following examples show how to do equivalent measure conversions.

You say pounds, I say kilograms.

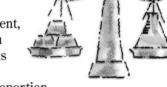

To prepare medications for your hypotensive patient, you must determine her weight in kilograms. You know that she weighs 125 lb, but how much is this in kilograms? Here's how to find out:
• You know that 1 kg equals 2.2 lb. So set up a proportion using X as the unknown weight:

$$\frac{X \text{ kg}}{125 \text{ lb}} = \frac{1 \text{ kg}}{2.2 \text{ lb}}$$

• Cross-multiply the fractions:

$$X \text{ kg} \times 2.2 \text{ lb} = 1 \text{ kg} \times 125 \text{ lb}$$

• Find X by dividing both sides of the equation by 2.2 lb and canceling units that appear in both the numerator and denominator:

$$\frac{X \text{ kg} \times 2.2 \text{ lb}}{2.2 \text{ lb}} = \frac{1 \text{ kg} \times 125 \text{ lb}}{2.2 \text{ lb}}$$

$$X = 56.8 \text{ kg}$$

Your patient weighs 56.8 kg.

You say milliliters, I say cups.

Your patient who's on a clear liquid diet must drink 480 ml of water for lunch. How many cups is this equal to? Here's how to find out:
• You know that 1 cup equals 240 ml. So set up a proportion using X as the unknown number:

$$\frac{X \text{ cups}}{480 \text{ ml}} = \frac{1 \text{ cup}}{240 \text{ ml}}$$

• Cross-multiply the fractions:

$$X \text{ cups} \times 240 \text{ ml} = 1 \text{ cup} \times 480 \text{ ml}$$

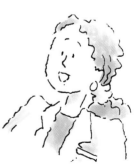

• Find X by dividing both sides of the equation by 240 ml and canceling units that appear in both the numerator and denominator:

$$\frac{X \text{ cups} \times 240 \text{ ml}}{240 \text{ ml}} = \frac{1 \text{ cup} \times 480 \text{ ml}}{240 \text{ ml}}$$

$$X = 2 \text{ cups}$$

Your patient needs to drink 2 cups of water.

You say tablespoons, I say milliliters.

The doctor orders 30 ml of milk of magnesia for your patient's heartburn. How many tablespoons is this? Here's how to find out:
• You know that 1 tbs contains 15 ml, so 2 tbs equal 30 ml.
• You can do this calculation in your head without setting up a proportion. Your patient had 2 tbs of milk of magnesia.

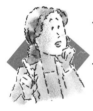

Quick quiz

1. The Arabic numeral 575 in Roman numerals is:
   A. DXXXXXXXV
   B. DLXXV
   C. CCCCCLXXV

Answer: B. To convert 575, break it into its component parts (500, 70, and 5); then translate the parts into Roman numerals.

2. The symbol ss represents:
   A. one-half.
   B. the abbreviation for "without."
   C. the dram symbol.

Answer: A. The symbol ss represents one-half in Roman numerals.

3. Drugs that are measured in units include:
   A. penicillin V, insulin, and heparin.
   B. co-trimoxazole.
   C. cough medicine.

Answer: A. Co-trimoxazole is measured in milligrams and cough medicine is commonly measured in teaspoons.

4. Electrolytes are measured in:
   A. grains.
   B. milligrams.
   C. milliequivalents.

Answer: C. Most electrolytes, like potassium chloride, are measured in milliequivalents.

5. When converting pounds to kilograms you should:
   A   multiply by 2.54
   B. divide by 2.2
   C. divide by 2.54

Answer: B. One kilogram equals 2.2 lb. By dividing pounds by 2.2, you obtain kilograms.

6. Before the metric system was established, doctors and pharmacists used the:
   A. apothecaries' system.
   B. avoirdupois system.
   C. household system.

Answer: A. Used before the metric system, the apothecaries' system is being phased out today.

7. The abbreviation for teaspoon is:
   A. tbs
   B. tsp
   C. t

Answer: B. The appropriate abbreviation is tsp. Don't use "t" — it's easy to misinterpret when written quickly.

8. The equivalent in milliliters of 55 U of NPH insulin (U-100) is:
   A. 55 ml
   B. 0.55 ml
   C. 5 ml

Answer: B. To do the conversion, set up the proportion:

$$\frac{X \, \text{ml}}{55 \, \text{U}} = \frac{1 \, \text{ml}}{100 \, \text{U}}$$

Cross-multiply the fractions, then divide both sides of the equation by 100 U and cancel units that appear in both the numerator and denominator to get 0.55 ml:

$$\frac{X \text{ ml} \times \cancel{100\ U}}{\cancel{100\ U}} = \frac{1 \text{ ml} \times 55 \cancel{U}}{100 \cancel{U}}$$

$$X = 0.55 \text{ ml}$$

9. The equivalent of 1 tsp of medication in milliliters is:
    A. 15 or 16 ml
    B. 4 or 5 ml
    C. 30 or 32 ml

Answer: B. 1 tsp equals 4 or 5 ml.

Scoring

☆☆☆ If you answered all nine items correctly, fantastic! Reward yourself with a minim of ice cream (alright, you can have a pint).

☆☆ If you answered six to eight correctly, good job! Have a fluid dram of champagne (enjoy every minim!).

☆ If you answered fewer than six correctly, keep at it. In the meantime, have a dram of chocolate (savor every grain!).

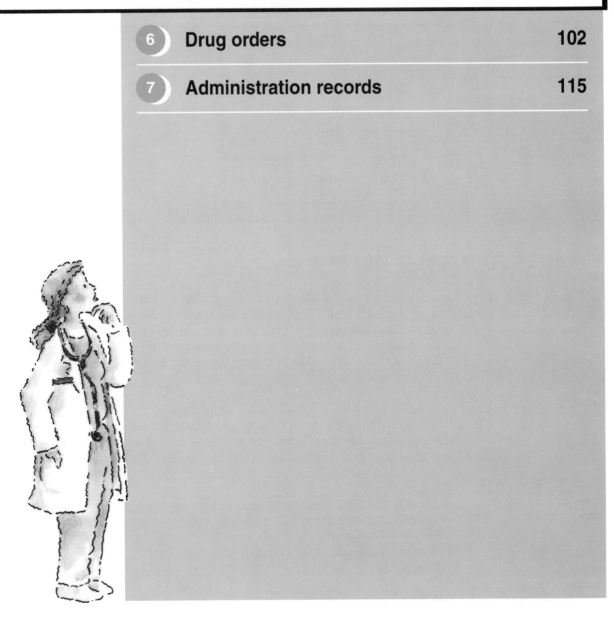

Part III

Recording drug administration

Drug orders

Just the facts

In this chapter, you'll learn:

♦ what a drug order consists of

♦ how to interpret drug orders using standard abbreviations

♦ how to use military time

♦ how to avoid making drug administration errors

♦ what to do about unclear drug orders.

A look at drug orders

Administering drugs is one of your most critical nursing responsibilities. It's also the area with the smallest margin for error. How can you prevent drug errors? The best way is by knowing how to read and correctly interpret drug orders. To do this, you need to understand what a drug order is and how it's used.

Direct handoff

In an outpatient setting, a doctor or health care professional who's licensed to prescribe drugs writes an order on a prescription form and gives it directly to the patient.

Keyboard, form, or fax

The routine for administering drugs is different for inpatient facilities. There, the doctor generates a drug order in one of the following ways:
• by entering the order into a computer system, which transmits it to the pharmacy and to the nurses' station

• by writing the order on the drug order sheet in the patient's chart

• by faxing the order to a pharmacy. (This method saves time by preventing an order from sitting in a patient's chart or computer before it's checked. However, the patient's confidentiality may be breached by this method.)

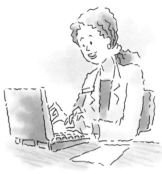

What's in a drug order?

The drug order sheet in a patient's chart must include all patient information, so it's usually stamped with the patient's admission data plate. When writing the order, the doctor includes all of the following:

• date and time of the order

• name of the drug, either generic or trade

• dosage form in metric, apothecaries', or household measurements

• abbreviation for the route of administration, such as P.O., I.M., S.C., I.V., P.R., P.V., or S.L. (In some health care facilities, if the route isn't specified, the oral route may be assumed.)

• administration schedule written as times per day or as number of hours between doses

• restrictions or specifications related to the order

• doctor's signature or name and code number in a computerized system (One signature or name and code number is sufficient after a group of orders.)

• doctor's registration number for controlled drugs, if applicable.

Write orders as ordered

Standard guidelines exist for writing drug orders. Being aware of these guidelines will help you interpret drug orders:

• The generic name of a drug is written entirely in lower-case letters.

• The trade or brand name of a drug begins with a capital letter.

• Drug abbreviations are written entirely in capital letters; however, drug names usually aren't abbreviated.

• Write information in this sequence: drug name, dosage, administration route, and time and frequency of administration.

A brief bit about abbreviating

Standard abbreviations are used to describe drug measurements, dosages, routes and times of administration, and related terms. The Joint Commission on Accreditation of Healthcare Organizations requires every health care facility to develop a list of approved abbreviations for staff use. (See *Making it short and sweet,* pages 105 and 106.)

Remember that abbreviations can easily be misinterpreted, especially if they're written carelessly or quickly. If one seems unusual or doesn't make sense to you, contact the doctor for clarification. Then clearly write out the correct term in your revision and transcription.

Marching in time (military time, that is)

Some doctors and health care facilities require pharmacologic orders and medication administration records to be written and transcribed in military time. (See *Military time,* page 107.) For example, an order might read *Lasix 40 mg I.V. b.i.d. at 0900 and 2100 hours.*

Simply confusing or confusingly simple?

Military time might seem confusing at first, but it's actually simple to use. This method of time is based on a 24-hour system. Here's how it works:

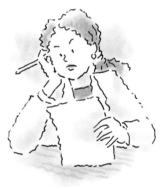

• To write single-digit times between 1:00 a.m. and 12:59 p.m., put a zero before the times and remove the colon. For example, 1:00 a.m. is written 0100 hours.
• To write double-digit times between 1:00 a.m. and 12:59 p.m., just remove the colon. For example, 11:00 a.m. becomes 1100 hours.
• The minutes after the hour remain the same. For example, 4:45 a.m. becomes 0445 hours.
• To write times from 1:00 p.m. to 12 midnight, simply add 1200 to the hour and remove the colon. For example, 1:00 p.m. becomes 1300 hours (1:00 + 12:00); 3:30 p.m. becomes 1530 hours (3:30 + 12:00); and 12:00 a.m (midnight) becomes 2400 hours (12:00 + 12:00).
• To write the minutes between 12:01 a.m. and 12:59 a.m., start over with zero. For example, 12:33 a.m. becomes 0033 hours.

Making it short and sweet

Standard abbreviations are handy for quickly and accurately transcribing medication orders and documenting drug administration. Use these abbreviations for drug measurements, dosage forms, routes and times of administration, and related terms.

Drug and solution measurements

cc	cubic centimeter
fl dr	fluid dram
fl oz	fluid ounce
g	gram
gal	gallon
gr	grain
gtt	drop
kg	kilogram
L	liter
mcg	microgram

Drug dosage forms

cap	capsule
DS	double strength
elix	elixir
LA	long-acting
liq	liquid
SA	sustained action
SR	sustained release
sol	solution

Routes of drug administration

A.D.	right ear
A.S.	left ear
A.U	each ear
I.M.	intramuscular
NG tube	nasogastric tube
O.D.	right eye

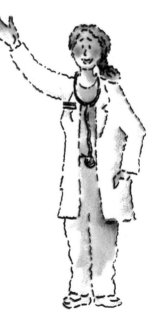

(continued)

Making it short and sweet *(continued)*

Routes of drug administration *(continued)*

O.S	left eye
O.U.	each eye
P.O. or p.o.	by mouth
P.V.	vaginally
S.C.	subcutaneous
S.L.	sublingually

Times of drug administration

a.c.	before meals
b.i.d.	twice a day
h.s.	at bedtime
p.c.	after meals
p.r.n.	as needed
q.a.m.	every morning
q.d.	every day
q.o.d.	every other day
q4h	every four hours

Miscellaneous abbreviations

AMA	against medical advice
ASAP	as soon as possible
BP	blood pressure
BPM	breaths per minute
c̄	with
D/C or dc	discontinue
KVO	keep vein open
MR	may repeat
NKA	no known allergies
NPO	nothing by mouth
<	less than
>	greater than
sys	systolic

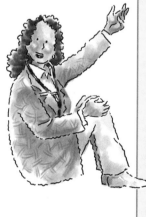

Dealing with drug orders

Once you determine that a drug order contains all the necessary information, you can begin to interpret it. (See *Say it in English,* page 108.) Read on to find guidelines for dealing with illegible handwriting, timing drug administration, renewing drug orders, and discontinued drug orders.

Hospital hieroglyphics

If any required information is missing, or if the doctor's handwriting is illegible, check with the doctor and clarify the order before signing the transcription. Also ask the doctor for clarification if nonstandard abbreviations are used.

Once the order is clear, sign it and send a contact copy or carbon copy to the pharmacy, where the drug will be dispensed according to your facility's policy.

Calibrating the clinical clock

Although the drug order sheet tells you when to give a drug, the actual administration time depends on three things:

Military time

Study the two clocks below to better understand military time. The clock on the left represents the hours from 1 a.m. (0100 hours) to noon (1200 hours). The clock on the right represents the hours from 1 p.m. (1300 hours) to midnight (2400 hours).

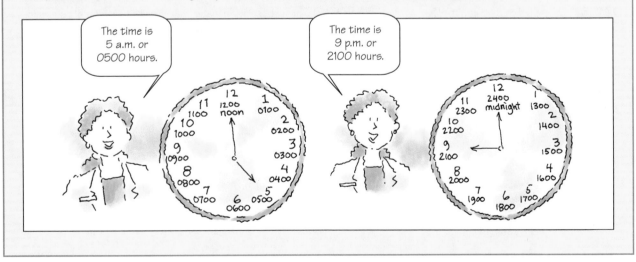

• your facility's policy (for drugs that are given a specific number of times per day)
• the nature of the drug
• the drug's onset and duration of action.

Say it in English

The following examples illustrate how to read and interpret a wide range of drug orders.

Drug order	Interpretation
Colace 100 mg P.O. b.i.d. p.c.	Give 100 mg of Colace by mouth twice a day after meals.
Vistaril 25 mg I.M. q3h p.r.n.	Give 25 mg of Vistaril intramuscularly every 3 hours, as needed.
Increase Duramorph to 6 mg I.V. q8h	Increase Duramorph to 6 mg intravenously every 8 hours.
folic acid 1 mg P.O. q.d.	Give 1 mg of folic acid by mouth daily.
Minipress 4 mg P.O. q6h, hold for sys BP < 120	Give 4 mg of Minipress by mouth every 6 hours; withhold drug if the systolic blood pressure falls below 120 mm Hg.
nifedipine 30 mg S.L. q4h	Give 30 mg of nifedipine sublingually every 4 hours.
Begin aspirin 325 mg P.O. q.d.	Begin giving 325 mg of aspirin by mouth daily.
Persantine 75 mg P.O. t.i.d.	Give 75 mg of Persantine by mouth three times a day.
aspirin grains v P.O. t.i.d.	Give 5 grains of aspirin by mouth three times a day.
Vasotec 2.5 mg P.O. q.d.	Give 2.5 mg of Vasotec by mouth daily.
1,000 ml D_5W c̄ KCl 20 mEq I.V. at 100 ml/h	Give 1,000 ml of dextrose 5% in water with 20 milliequivalents of potassium chloride intravenously at a rate of 100 milliliters per hour.
D/C penicillin I.V., start penicillin G 800,000 U P.O. q6h	Discontinue intravenous penicillin; start 800,000 units of penicillin G by mouth every 6 hours.
diphenhydramine 25–50 mg P.O. h.s. p.r.n.	Give 25 to 50 mg of diphenhydramine by mouth at bedtime, as needed.

Short-winded

Persantine 75 mg P.O. t.i.d.

Give 75 mg of Persantine by mouth three times a day.

Long-winded

Be sure to administer drugs within one-half hour of the times specified on the drug order sheet.

After giving a drug, record the actual time of administration on the medication administration record.

Reevaluate, renew, reorder

Health care facilities also have policies for how often drug orders must be renewed. For example, narcotics may need to be reordered every 24, 48, or 72 hours. This allows health care professionals to reevaluate the patient's need for the drug and to adjust the dosage or frequency of administration, if necessary.

Remember that I.V. fluids—such as normal saline solution, dextrose and water, and hyperalimentation or total parenteral nutrition solutions—are considered drugs. Check all I.V. fluid orders carefully. Most health care facilities provide guidelines for the renewal of I.V. fluids as well as for other drugs.

Stop! That's an order.

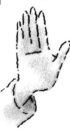

If the doctor decides to discontinue a drug before the original order runs out, he must write a new order. These orders also must be precise.

For example, if an order reads *D/C K* and the patient is receiving vitamin K and potassium chloride, you'll need to contact the doctor to clarify which medication he wants to discontinue.

Handling ambiguous drug orders

All too often, drug orders are unclear because of nonstandard abbreviations, illegible handwriting, incorrect dosages, or missing information. It helps if handwritten orders are neat, with drugs spelled correctly. (See *Don't struggle with difficult orders*, page 110.)

Rule #1: Never trust a computer

Even if the doctor enters drug orders into the computer system, your interpretation skills are still extremely important. Although computers solve the problem of illegible handwriting, they can't correct human error. A computer will accept the wrong drug, the wrong dose, the wrong route, and the wrong frequency.

Before you give that drug

Don't struggle with difficult orders

The combination of poor handwriting and inappropriate abbreviations on a drug order can lead to confusion and medication errors. Have the doctor clarify an order that's difficult to understand or that seems wrong.

If you can't read something on the drug order, ask the doctor for clarification.

FREEDOM HOSPITAL

UNIT NO. 4 SOUTH, 432A
NAME JOE JACKSON
ADDRESS 33 SHORT STREET
CITY HOPE, NJ BIRTH 2·21·24

DOCTOR'S ORDERS
INSTRUCTIONS
1. Each time a physicians writes a medication order, detach top copy and send to pharmacy.
2. Rule off unused lines after last copy (Pink) has been sent to pharmacy.
DO NOT USE THIS SHEET
UNLESS A NUMBER SHOWS.

1

DATE	TIME	ORDERS	DOCTOR'S SIGNATURE	NURSE'S SIGNATURE
2/14	12³⁰ p			

Discharge diagnoses in order of decreasing priority must be supplied at time of patient's discharge.

Rule #2: Advocate appropriate administration

Your responsibility in interpreting orders includes making sure that the ordered drug is an appropriate treatment. This is where your role as patient advocate comes in. To make sure the drug you're asked to administer is appropriate, do the following:

• Think critically; don't be timid about asking for clarification and justification.

• Know the action of each drug you give and the purpose for which it's given.

• If a drug order seems questionable, use all available resources to check it. For example, ask the doctor, the pharmacist, and your colleagues, and refer to a drug handbook.

• Always check the five "rights" before giving a drug. (See *Do the right thing*.)

• Check and recheck all your drug calculations.

• Never administer a drug that's improperly labeled or that you personally didn't draw from a vial.

• Never use open or unmarked I.V. solution bags.

Practice with poorly written orders

The following are examples of poorly written drug orders that need to be clarified by the doctor who wrote them. See if you can find the errors.

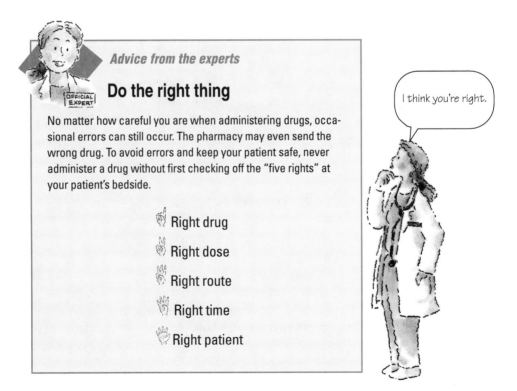

Advice from the experts

Do the right thing

No matter how careful you are when administering drugs, occasional errors can still occur. The pharmacy may even send the wrong drug. To avoid errors and keep your patient safe, never administer a drug without first checking off the "five rights" at your patient's bedside.

Right drug

Right dose

Right route

Right time

Right patient

I think you're right.

Whadd'ya want?

K 40 mEq I.V. q.d. —the drug being ordered is unclear. Is it vitamin K or potassium chloride (KCl)? If it's KCl, remember that this electrolyte must be diluted in I.V. fluid before administration.

How d'ya want it?

Digoxin 0.25 mg q.d. —the administration route is missing. Digoxin may be given orally as a pill or elixir or I.V.

When d'ya want it?

Nifedipine 10 mg S.L. —the frequency of administration is missing. Nifedipine can be given in a single dose for hypertension, or it can be given on another schedule as a maintenance drug. In the latter case, it's usually given orally.

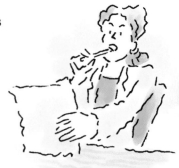

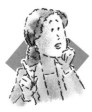

Quick quiz

1. Drug abbreviations should be written:
    A.   in lowercase letters.
    B.   in capital letters.
    C.   with the first letter in capitals.

Answer: B. Drug abbreviations should be avoided, but when they're used they should be in all capital letters.

2. The correct abbreviation for after meals is:
    A.   P.O.
    B.   P.R.
    C.   p.c.

Answer: C. P.O. stands for by mouth, and P.R. stands for by rectum.

3. The abbreviation MR stands for:
    A.   milligram.
    B.   may repeat.
    C.   may remove.

Answer: B. Milligram is abbreviated mg, and may remove has no standard abbreviation.

4. The order *morphine 4 mg I.M. q4h p.r.n. pain, hold for respiratory rate < 12 BPM* means:
   A. give morphine 4 mg intramuscularly 4 times a day for pain, hold for respiratory rate less than 12 breaths per minute.
   B. give morphine 4 mg intramuscularly every 4 hours for pain, hold for respiratory rate greater than 12 breaths per minute.
   C. give morphine 4 mg intramuscularly every 4 hours as needed for pain, hold for respiratory rate less than 12 breaths per minute.

Answer: C. Every 4 hours is abbreviated q4h, the abbreviation p.r.n. means as needed, and the symbol < means less than.

5. In military time, 3:08 p.m. is:
   A. 308 hours.
   B. 1508 hours.
   C. 1308 hours.

Answer: B. To convert a time between 1:00 p.m. and 12:00 midnight, remove the colon and add the number to 1200 hours.

6. "Give Dilantin 150 mg by mouth twice a day at 0900 hours and 2100 hours, draw Dilantin levels every other day" can be written on a drug order as:
   A. *Dilantin 150 mg P.O. b.i.d at 9:00 a.m. and 9:00 p.m., draw Dilantin levels q.o.d.*
   B. *Dilantin 150 mg P.O. t.i.d. at 9:00 a.m. and 9:00 p.m., draw Dilantin levels q.d.*
   C. *Dilantin 150 mp I.V. b.i.d. at 9:00 a.m. and 9:00 p.m., draw Dilantin levels q.o.d.*

Answer: A. In answer B, t.i.d. means three times a day, and q.d. means every day. In answer C, mp isn't a standard abbreviation, and I.V. means intravenous.

7. Using a computer to order drugs:
   A. decreases patient confidentiality.
   B. helps pinpoint errors in writing orders.
   C. solves the problem of illegible handwriting.
Answer: C. A computer can make orders legible, but it can't spot errors.

8. The five "rights" of drug administration are:
   A. drug, dose, route, time, patient.
   B. drug, filter, solution, doctor, shift.
   C. drug, order, signature, time, patient.

Answer: A. To help ensure patient safety, go through this checklist before administering a drug.

Scoring

☆☆☆   If you answered all eight items correctly, wow! You're error-free!

☆☆   If you answered five to seven correctly, you're almost there! You can spot an incorrect order, recognize standard abbreviations, and read hospital hieroglyphics!

☆   If you answered fewer than five correctly, keep going! You're acquiring the art of the drug order!

Administration records

Just the facts

In this chapter, you'll learn:

♦ what types of administration record systems are used

♦ how to document on the administration record

♦ how to prevent drug errors

♦ how to report drug errors.

A look at administration records

Maintaining accurate medication administration records is a vital nursing responsibility, both for legal reasons and for patient safety. The liability risk of the health care provider may increase if medication administration isn't properly documented. In terms of patient safety, documentation that's missing or inaccurate can lead to drug errors that can jeopardize your patient's health.

Record-keeping systems

Three main types of medication administration record systems are in use today: the Kardex, the medication administration record (MAR), and computer charting.

Don't get unhinged

Some units use the Kardex system, which consists of a set of large index cards in a hinged file. The file is usually kept in the medication room or on the medication cart, although individual cards also may be clipped to the patient's chart or clipboard.

Charts on MARs

Another widely used system, the MAR, is an $8\frac{1}{2}'' \times 11''$ form that goes into the patient's chart. (Some units use a combination of both the Kardex and the MAR.)

Charting on-line

A third system, computer charting, is being used by more and more health care facilities. Information is entered into a computer, which automatically generates a list of administration times for all scheduled medications. Computer systems cut the risk of drug errors caused by illegible handwriting. (See *Record keeping in the computer age.*)

See you in court

No matter what type of medication charting system your facility uses, you must still record certain standard information. (See *Different forms, same info,* page 118.) Standardization allows medication administration records to be used as legal documents if it ever becomes necessary to prove that a drug dose was given.

Documentation

In general, documentation reflects the tasks, assessments, and procedures nurses perform. Documenting on the administration record indicates that you've carried out the doctor's order.

Does that say subcutaneous or subcuticular?

Before transcribing the doctor's orders, make sure that they're complete, clear, and correct. If you detect a problem, contact the doctor before sending the order to the pharmacy. If the order goes to the pharmacy and then you detect a problem, contact both the doctor and the pharmacy.

Is that 1 mg I.V. over 10 minutes or 10 mg over 1 minute?

Information recorded on a Kardex or MAR must be written legibly in ink. All handwritten or computerized administration records must contain patient information, drug information, and signatures. *Remember: Transcribing drug orders requires close attention because even a small discrepancy can cause a major drug error.*

Recording patient information

If your institution uses a computerized system, you don't need to transcribe patient information onto the administration record. It's already there because the admissions office enters the patient information into the system and the

---

Record keeping in the computer age

As health care facilities purchase or develop computer systems, manufacturers offer increased choices among medication monitoring programs.

From simple...
Computerized record systems range from simple to sophisticated. In the simplest systems, the computer is used as a word processor or typewriter.

...To sophisticated
In more sophisticated systems, doctors can order drugs from the pharmacy by typing the drug's name or by selecting specific drugs by searching through various listings, such as pharmacologic categories, pharmacokinetic categories, and disease-related uses.

The computer indicates whether the pharmacy has the drug. The order then goes into the pharmacy's computer for filling. The order also generates the patient's record, on which the nurse can document medication administration.

Benefits bit by bit
Computer systems offer the following advantages:

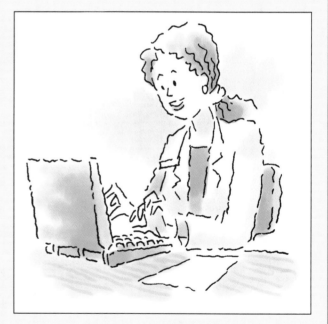

• When drug orders are changed, the pharmacy receives immediate notification, so drugs arrive on the unit faster.
• The pharmacy's computer can immediately confirm or deny a drug's availability.
• Nurses can document on medication records quickly and easily.
• Nurses can see at a glance which drugs have already been administered and which still need to be.
• Errors from misinterpreted handwriting are eliminated.
• Records can be stored on disk in addition to, or instead of, paper copies.

pharmacy adds information, such as the patient's height, weight, and allergies. If you use a Kardex or MAR, stamp the form with the patient's admission data plate. If this isn't available, copy the information from the patient's identification bracelet.

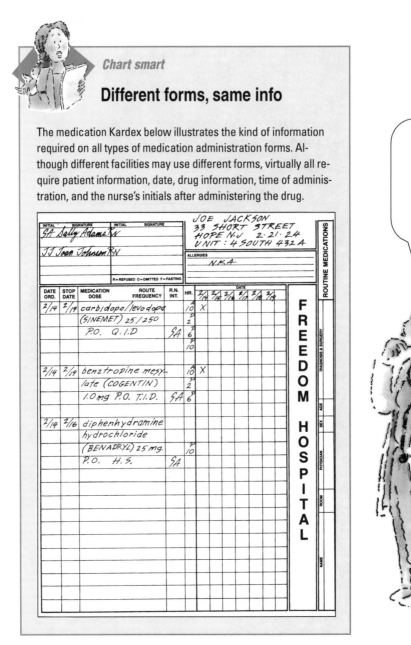

Chart smart

Different forms, same info

The medication Kardex below illustrates the kind of information required on all types of medication administration forms. Although different facilities may use different forms, virtually all require patient information, date, drug information, time of administration, and the nurse's initials after administering the drug.

No matter what form is used, I have to make sure all the info is there!

Identification, please

Record the patient's full name, hospital identification number, unit number, bed assignment, and allergies, even those that aren't drug related. If the patient doesn't have any known allergies, write "NKA."

If the name of his insurance carrier is written on his identification bracelet, record this, too. *Transcribe the information exactly as it appears on the bracelet.*

Recording drug information

Next, transcribe from the doctor's order complete information about every drug the patient is taking. Include dates and drug names, dosages, strengths, dosage forms, administration routes, and administration times.

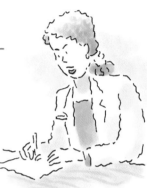

It's a date!

You must always record these dates on the administration record: the date the prescription was written; the date the drug should begin, if this is different from the original order date; and the date the drug should be discontinued.

Even more precise

At some facilities, the time and date the drug should begin are recorded together. This serves as a reference for the time to discontinue a drug when a limited period is indicated. Many facilities also have a standard length of time a drug may be given before it's automatically discontinued.

Full name, please

Record the drug's full generic name. If the doctor ordered the drug using a proprietary name, record this name as well. Don't use abbreviations, chemical symbols, research names, or special facility names. This can cause medication errors or a delay in therapy.

Dose and strength

When recording drug strength, be sure to write the actual amount of the drug to be administered. If the dose you administer varies in any way from the strength or amount ordered, note this in a special area on the administration record if there is one or in the patient's progress notes.

For example, document whether the patient refused to take a drug, consumed only part of a drug, or vomited shortly after taking a drug.

Proper form

Also record the drug dosage form that the doctor ordered. Then decide whether the form is appropriate, considering the patient's special needs.

For example, if sustained-action theophylline tablets are ordered for a patient with a nasogastric tube, he won't be able to take the tablets orally. You'll have to crush them before administering them through the tube.

However, crushing sustained-action tablets destroys the drug's integrity and alters its therapeutic action. So, you'll need to contact the doctor and discuss an alternative drug dosage form.

The route of the matter

Recording the route of administration is especially critical for drugs that may be given by two different routes. For example, acetaminophen can be given orally or rectally. Other drugs can be given by only one correct route; for example, NPH insulin may be given subcutaneously but not intravenously.

Citing the site

When administering a drug by a parenteral, intramuscular, or subcutaneous route, record the injection site to facilitate site rotation. Most administration forms include a numbered list of recognized sites, allowing you to record the site by its number.

If you administer a drug by a different route than the route the doctor originally ordered, indicate that change, along with the reason and authorization for the change.

Schedule scheme

The doctor's order should include an administration schedule, such as t.i.d. or q6h. Transcribe the schedule onto the administration record, and then convert it into actual times based on your facility's policy and the drug's availability, characteristics, onset, and duration of action.

For example, t.i.d. may mean 9 a.m., 1 p.m., and 5 p.m. in one facility, and 10 a.m., 2 p.m., and 6 p.m. in another. And b.i.d. may be 10 a.m. and 6 p.m. or 10 a.m. and 10 p.m.

Be sure to record the drug dosage form.

'Round the clock (the 24-hour clock, that is)

Remember that time notations are based on a 24-hour clock, unless otherwise specified. This means that the hour appearing first on a 24-hour clock should appear first in the time notation.

In other words, if an administration schedule is 2-10-2-10, the first 2 represents 2 a.m., or 0200 hours; the first 10 represents 10 a.m., or 1000 hours; the second 2 is 2 p.m., or 1400 hours; and the second 10 is 10 p.m., or 2200 hours.

Special space

Some facilities have separate administration records or specially designated areas of the regular administration record for recording single orders or special drug orders. Special orders include drugs given p.r.n., large-volume parenteral drugs, and dermatologic and ophthalmic medications dispensed in bottles or tubes.

Other facilities put single orders or special drugs on the regular administration record. If this is the case where you work, be very careful to distinguish these drugs from regularly scheduled ones. All facilities have special forms for recording controlled substances. (See *Controlling controlled substances*.)

Time check

Immediately after giving a drug, document the time of administration to keep you from mistakenly giving the drug again. For scheduled drugs, you'll usually initial the appropriate time slot for the date that the drug is administered.

Fashionably late

Scheduled drugs are considered on time if they're given one-half hour before or after the ordered time. For unscheduled drugs, such as single doses or p.r.n. drugs, record the exact time of administration in the appropriate slot.

Unfashionably late

If you don't give a drug on time, or if you miss a dose, document the reason why on either the administration record or the patient's progress notes. Facility policy may require you to initial and circle the particular time missed on the administration record to draw attention to it.

Controlling controlled substances

Federal and state laws regulate the dispensing, administering, and documenting of controlled substances. When these substances are issued to a unit, they're accompanied by a perpetual inventory record.

A paper trail
If the doctor orders a controlled substance for your patient, record its administration on the administration record and the perpetual inventory record. When you remove a dose from the locked storage site, record this information on the perpetual inventory record:
• date and time the dose is removed
• patient's full name
• doctor's name
• drug dose
• your signature.

If you have to discard any of the dose, have another nurse verify the amount discarded and sign the form, too.

Signature, please

Every time you document on the administration record, you must sign it. First, initial the record after transcribing from the doctor's order sheet. Many facilities also require the nurse to perform a chart check and initial the doctor's order sheet on a line after the last order. This indicates that all orders have been transcribed correctly onto the administration record.

If someone other than a nurse transcribes the order, a nurse must co-sign the order sheet and the administration record.

Monogram mania

You also need to sign the administration record after giving a drug. Put your initials in the appropriate space on the form. Be sure they're legible, and always sign them the same way. If another nurse on your unit has the same initials, use your middle initial to avoid confusion.

In addition, write your full name, title, and initials in the signature section of the administration record. This information must appear on every record that you initial when administering drugs.

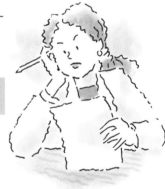

Assuring quality and preventing errors

Each facility has its own method for tracking errors in drug administration. Unfortunately, many errors aren't documented because the administering nurse is afraid to report them. But tracking and documenting errors allows the quality assurance team to recommend ways to prevent them in the future and keep patients safe.

Eradicating errors

One way to decrease medication errors is by adhering to your facility's policies, suggested safety precautions, and quality assurance recommendations. Another way is by transcribing orders carefully from the doctor's order sheet to the administration record.

Sensible safeguards

To avoid transcription errors, follow these guidelines:

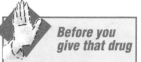

• Transcribe orders in a quiet area where you can concentrate without interruptions.
• Before signing the order sheet and initialing the administration record, carefully check both forms.
• Follow your facility's policy for reviewing orders. Some require nurses to check all patient charts for new orders several times each shift and also to check orders written within the last 24 hours. Other facilities give one shift, usually the night shift, this last responsibility.

Refusing to give a drug

On rare occasions, you may be asked to administer a drug that you feel uncomfortable with. You can legally refuse to administer a drug under these circumstances:
• if you think the dosage prescribed is too high
• if you think the drug might interact dangerously with other drugs the patient is taking or substances such as alcohol
• if you think the patient's physical condition contraindicates using the drug.

The right way to say no

When you refuse to carry out a drug order, be sure you do the following:
• Notify your immediate supervisor so she can make alternative arrangements (assigning a new nurse, clarifying the order).
• Notify the prescribing doctor if your supervisor hasn't done so already.
• If your employer requires it, document that the drug wasn't given and explain why.

Easy does it

Many drug errors occur because nurses are in a hurry or are unfamiliar with a drug. Try to take your time. Remember that many drugs are derivatives of other drugs, so they have similar names. (See *Conquering confusion.*) If a drug is new to you, use available resources to find out all you can about it.

Before you give that drug

Conquering confusion

Before giving a drug, remind yourself of these essential tactics.

Remember the rights
Check off the five "rights"—right drug, right dose, right route, right time, and right patient.

Look at the label
Examine drug labels closely — many of them look alike.

Notice the name
Pay attention! Many drugs have similar-sounding names. Consider the examples below:
• interferon and Imferon
• Compazine and Thorazine
• hydromorphone and morphine
• Pavulon and Parafon
• cefoxitin and Ceftin.

Reporting drug errors

Even though you take precautions, you may still make a drug error. Or, you may administer a drug correctly, only to have a patient react negatively to it. When this happens, the value of meticulous documentation becomes clear.

A rational response

If an error occurs, follow these steps:
• Notify the doctor immediately.
• Consult the pharmacist. He can provide information about drug interactions, dose-related problems such as what to do about an overdose or an omitted dose, and an antidote, if needed.
• Continue to assess the patient, paying close attention to the drug's action and possible effects.
• Follow your facility's policy for documenting drug errors. You may have to complete an incident report for legal purposes. If so, clearly document what happened without defending an action or placing blame. Record the names and functions of everyone involved and what actions you all took to protect the patient after the error was discovered.

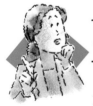

Quick quiz

1. You may be required to circle and initial the time slot of a medication if:
    A. you missed the dose or gave it late.
    B. the administration time has changed.
    C. another nurse forgot to administer a drug.

Answer: A. Circling and initialing the time slot signals to the next nurse that the dose was missed or late. The nurse then refers to the single order or PRN section of the MAR to find the actual administration time. This way, she doesn't mistakenly administer the next dose too soon.

2. The information on the patient's admission data plate is:
    A. full name, social security number, birth date, and

doctor's name.
B. full name, hospital identification number, bed location, unit number, and allergies.
C. full name, address, and doctor's name.

Answer: B. The patient's address and insurance company name also may appear on the plate.

3. Injection site rotation is facilitated when each nurse documents:
A. the time of the last injection.
B. the date of the last injection.
C. the site of the last injection.

Answer: C. Recording the site tells the next nurse what sites have already been used so she doesn't repeat them.

4. You have the right to refuse to administer a drug if:
A. you don't trust the doctor.
B. you think the dose is too high.
C. it doesn't arrive on time to give it on schedule.

Answer: B. You can also refuse to administer a drug if it would interact dangerously with other drugs the patient is taking or if it's contraindicated for his physical condition.

5. When a computerized system is used, the admissions office enters patient information and the pharmacy adds:
A. care plan changes.
B. allergy alerts.
C. perpetual records.

Answer: B. The pharmacy also adds other information, such as the patient's height and weight.

6. To avoid confusion, nurses with the same initials should sign the administration record with:
A. their identification numbers.
B. a different-colored pen.
C. their middle initial.

Answer: C. Also, be sure to write legibly and always sign the same way.

7. You should transcribe orders:
A. in the patient's room.
B. at the nurses' station.
C. in a quiet area.

Answer: C. Transcribing in a quiet area without distractions will help you concentrate.

Scoring

☆☆☆ If you answered all seven items correctly, amazing! You've been voted best nurse at the Administration Academy Awards!

☆☆ If you answered five or six correctly, fantastic! Here's your Oscar for best supporting nurse!

☆ If you answered less than five correctly, keep your chin up! You're still a record setter!

Part IV

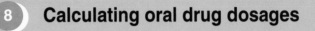

Oral, topical, and rectal drugs

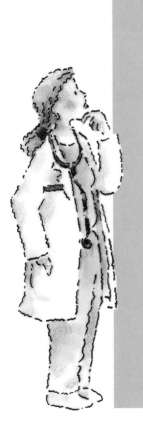

Calculating oral drug dosages

Just the facts

In this chapter, you'll learn:

♦ how to read drug labels to obtain accurate information for calculations

♦ how to administer drugs safely

♦ how to calculate oral dosages of tablets, capsules, and liquids

♦ how to calculate dosages using different measurement systems.

A look at oral drugs

Drugs that are administered by the oral route — through the mouth — are usually in tablet, capsule, or liquid form. Most oral drugs are available in a limited number of strengths or concentrations. Therefore, your ability to calculate prescribed dosages for various drug forms and strengths is an important skill.

Reading oral drug labels

Before you can administer an oral drug safely, you must be sure that it's the correct drug and the correct dose. Your first step is to read the label carefully, noting the drug's name, dose strength, and expiration date.

Drug name

When reading a drug label, check the generic name first. If the drug has two names, the generic name usually appears in smaller print. The generic name is the accepted nonproprietary name, which is a simplified form of the drug's chemical name.

Next, note the drug's trade name, also called the brand or proprietary name. This name, given by the manufacturer, usually appears first on the label, followed by the registration symbol.

Two in one

Some oral medications actually contain two different drugs. The labels for these combination drugs list both generic names and their doses. (See *A look at the label*.) These drugs are ordered by the trade name and the number of capsules or tablets or the volume of elixir to be given — for example, *Septra 1 tsp q12hr.*

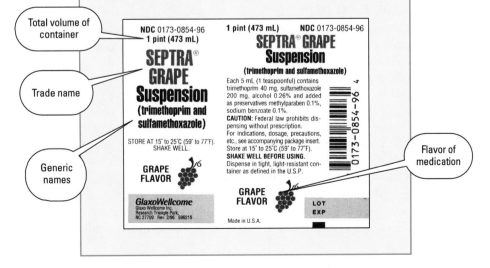

Before you give that drug

A look at the label

Before journeying into complex dosage computations, take a quick tour of this drug label. As this label states, Septra contains 40 mg of trimethoprim and 200 mg of sulfamethoxazole. So, instead of ordering it with a two-part dosage, the doctor prescribes it by the trade name Septra, and the volume of elixir to be given.

Total volume of container

Trade name

Generic names

Flavor of medication

NDC 0173-0854-96
1 pint (473 mL)

SEPTRA®
GRAPE
Suspension
(trimethoprim and sulfamethoxazole)

STORE AT 15° to 25°C (59° to 77°F).
SHAKE WELL.

GRAPE
FLAVOR

GlaxoWellcome
Glaxo Wellcome Inc.
Research Triangle Park,
NC 27709   Rev. 2/96   596215

1 pint (473 mL)   NDC 0173-0854-96

SEPTRA® GRAPE
Suspension
(trimethoprim and sulfamethoxazole)

Each 5 mL (1 teaspoonful) contains trimethoprim 40 mg, sulfamethoxazole 200 mg, alcohol 0.26% and added as preservatives methylparaben 0.1%, sodium benzoate 0.1%.
CAUTION: Federal law prohibits dispensing without prescription.
For indications, dosage, precautions, etc., see accompanying package insert.
Store at 15° to 25°C (59° to 77°F).
SHAKE WELL BEFORE USING.
Dispense in tight, light-resistant container as defined in the U.S.P.

GRAPE
FLAVOR

LOT
EXP

Made in U.S.A.

0173-0854-96 4

The name game

A drug may have several trade names, but it has only one generic name. For example, the generic drug diazepam goes by the trade names D-Val, Valium, Valrelease, Vazepam, and Zetran.

However, some drugs are so widely used and so well known by their generic names that the manufacturer never gives them a trade name. One example is atropine sulfate.

Meeting the standard

The initials U.S.P. or N.F. may appear after the drug name. They stand for two legally recognized standards for drugs: United States Pharmacopeia and National Formulary. These initials mean that a drug has met standards of purity, potency, and storage, which are enforced by the Food and Drug Administration.

Dose strength

After checking the drug name, look for the dose strength on the label. Pay close attention: The labels and containers for different concentrations of the same drug may look exactly alike except for the listing of the drug's concentration. (See *Look-alike labels: Tablets and capsules.*) The same goes for oral solutions. The labels can look similar for different concentrations of the same drug. (See *Look-alike labels: Oral solutions*, page 132.)

Expiration date

Finally, check the expiration date. This vital information is often overlooked. Expired drugs may be chemically unstable and may no longer provide the correct dose. If a drug has expired, return it to the pharmacy for proper disposal and so the patient can be reimbursed.

Administering oral drugs safely

The first rule in assuring the safest possible administration of drugs is to triple-check drug labels and drug orders. Safe drug administration requires you to compare the doctor's order — as transcribed on the medication administration record — against the drug label *three times*. (See *Say it three times: Check orders and labels*, page 133.)

Proceed with caution

The doctor has ordered *150 mg of ranitidine (Zantac) P.O.* for your patient. Before giving the drug, follow this procedure to the letter:

Before you give that drug

Look-alike labels: Tablets and capsules

Don't let yourself be lulled by look-alike labels. The following tablet and capsule labels are examples of look-alikes and sound-alikes that you must read carefully to avoid medication errors.

Norpramin and Norpace
On first glance, these medication names may be easily confused, which could lead to a medication error that could harm the patient. Norpramin is a tricyclic antidepressant, whereas Norpace is an antiarrhythmic. The inadvertent substitution of the antidepressant Norpramin for Norpace wouldn't control the patient's arrhythmia, which could lead to serious complications.

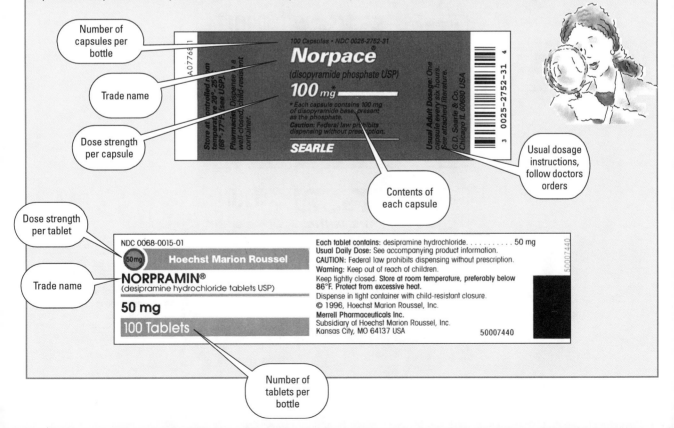

👆 Open the patient's medication drawer, find the drug labeled ranitidine (Zantac) 150 mg, and note that it's in oral tablet form.

✌️ Place the labeled drug next to the transcribed order on the administration record and carefully compare each part of the label to the order.

🤟 If the drug is supplied in bulk or in a stock bottle, transfer one tablet from the supply to a medication container, pouring from the supply to the lid and then into the container without handling the tablet.

Before you give that drug

Look-alike labels: Oral solutions

The oral solution labels below are examples of look-alikes that you are likely to encounter. Reading labels carefully can help you avoid medication errors.

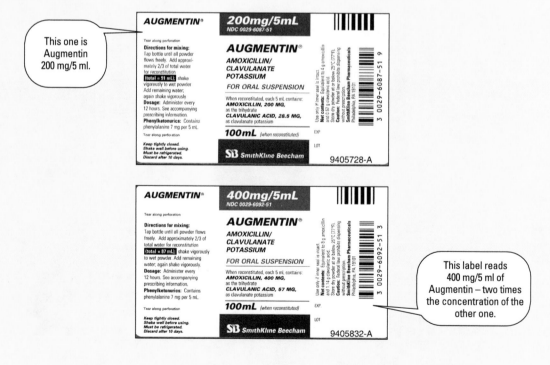

This one is Augmentin 200 mg/5 ml.

This label reads 400 mg/5 ml of Augmentin – two times the concentration of the other one.

Before returning the supply to the drawer or shelf, once again compare the label to the order on the administration record, again noting whether this is the right administration time. *Once you've removed a drug from its container, you can't ever be certain that it's the correct drug unless you have carefully compared the label to the administration record while pouring.*

Now, go to the patient's bedside, check his identification bracelet, and do your third drug check, comparing the label to the order and checking the administration time again. Then give the drug.

If the drug comes in a unit-dose packet, don't remove it from the packet until you're at the patient's bedside and ready to administer it. (See *Unit-dose packaging,* page 134.) Then do your third drug check. Remove the drug from the packet and give it to the patient, using the

Before you give that drug

Say it three times: Check orders and labels

The secret of drug safety is to check, check, and check again. Before giving a drug, carefully compare the drug's label with each part of the medication administration record, holding the label next to the administration record to ensure accuracy. The example below walks you through the steps for administering *furosemide (Lasix) 40 mg P.O.*

Check drug names
• Read the drug's generic name on the administration record, and compare it to the generic name on the label. They both should say *furosemide.*
• Read the trade name on the administration record, and compare it to the trade name on the label. They both should say *Lasix.*

Check dosage, route, and record
• Read the dosage on the administration record, and compare it to the dosage on the label. They both should say *40 mg.*
• Read the route specified on the administration record, and note the dosage form on the label. The record should say *P.O.* and the label should say *oral tablet.*

• Note any special considerations on the administration record, such as "aspiration precautions (head of bed elevated to 45 degrees for all P.O. intake);" "Patient is HOH (hard of hearing);" or "Patient is blind."

Check orders and labels three times
Follow this routine three times before giving the drug. Do it the first time when you obtain the drug from floor stock or the patient's supply. Do it the second time before placing the drug in the medication cup or other administration device. Finally, do it the third time before replacing the stock drug bottle on the shelf or removing the drug from the unit-dose packet at the patient's bedside.

Unit-dose packaging

Tablets or capsules in unit doses may be dispensed on a card with the drugs sealed in bubbles or in strips with each drug separated by a tear line. Unit doses of liquids may be packaged in small sealed cups with identifying information on the cover.

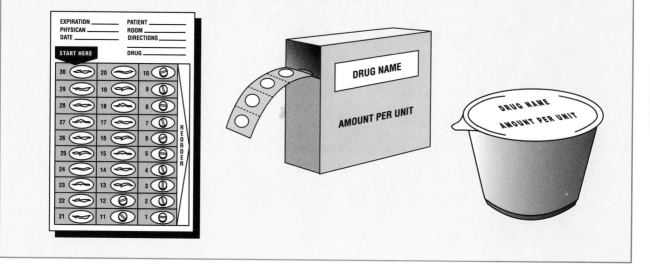

packet label for comparison when recording your administration information.

Discovering discrepancies

If you notice discrepancies between the administration record and the drug label, check them out. For example, suppose the administration record specifies Ceclor and the drug packet is labeled cefaclor. Check your drug handbook and you'll find out that Ceclor is a trade name for cefaclor.

Or, suppose the drug packet is labeled Ceclor 250 mg and the dose on the administration record is 500 mg. In this case, you need to calculate the required dose. Scrupulous attention to details like these will help ensure safe, error-free drug administration.

Unit-dose systems

Many institutions use the unit-dose system, which provides prepackaged drugs in single-dose containers and decreases the need for dosage calculations. (See *Save time with the unit-dose system.*)

Calculating dosages

Despite the prevalence of unit-dose systems, calculations are still necessary in many patient situations. For example, you may have to determine individualized dosages for special patients. You also must know how to convert between measurement systems to determine how many tablets, capsules, or other dosage forms to administer. (See *Special delivery drug dosages,* page 136.)

You'll often use ratios and fractions in proportions to calculate drug dosages and to convert between measurement systems. (See *Helpful hints to minimize math mistakes,* page 137.) The following section reviews these mathematical concepts and shows step-by-step calculations.

Using ratios, fractions, and proportions

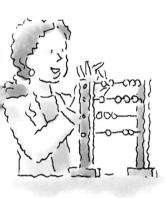

Ratios and fractions are two ways to express the numerical relationship between things. A proportion expresses equality between two ratios or fractions. Proportions may be written using ratios, as in

$$1:3::2:6$$

or using fractions, as in

$$\frac{1}{3} = \frac{2}{6}$$

When proportions are expressed using ratios, the product of the means, or the inside numbers, equals the product of the extremes, or the outside numbers:

$$\overset{\text{means}}{2:4}::\overset{}{1:2}$$
$$\underset{\text{extremes}}{}$$

so,

$$4 \times 1 = 2 \times 2$$

When proportions are expressed as fractions, their cross products are equal:

$$\frac{3}{6} \,\diagdown\!\!\!\!\diagup\, \frac{6}{12}$$

so,

$$3 \times 12 = 6 \times 6$$

Going to a mean extreme

When a proportion is expressed using ratios, the units of the mean on one side of the equal sign must match the units of the extreme on the other side, and vice versa:

$$mg : tablet :: mg : tablet$$

When a proportion is expressed using fractions, the units of measure in the numerators must be the same, and the units of measure in the denominators must be the same:

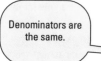

Denominators are the same.

$$\frac{mg}{tablet} = \frac{mg}{tablet}$$

Numerators are the same.

Four rules for calculating drug dosages

To help you prevent calculation and medication errors and to simplify your calculations, remember these four rules:

Special delivery drug dosages

Even if your facility uses the unit-dose system, you'll still need to calculate dosages for some patients. For example, patients on critical care units, pediatric patients, and geriatric patients required individualized medication dosages that may be unusually large or small.

The nearest milligram
Some patients need dosages that are calculated to the nearest milligram instead of the nearest 10 mg. For them, the correct calculation of the exact dosage can mean the difference between a drug underdose and an overdose. A few examples of drugs that are measured to the nearest milligram or microgram are digoxin, levothyroxine sodium, and many pediatric drugs.

Changing the delivery route
Some people just can't handle drugs that are delivered by the usual route because their ability to absorb, distribute, metabolize, or excrete drugs is impaired. Some patients can't ab-

sorb drugs from the GI tract because of upper GI disorders or surgery; deficiencies of gastric, pancreatic, or intestinal secretions; or passive congestion of GI blood vessels from severe congestive heart failure. These patients need drugs in parenteral form in larger-than-average oral doses. Drugs given I.V. may be in smaller doses because they may be delivered to the bloodstream more efficiently and are more readily absorbed.

Don't forget these special patients
Other patients who need individualized dosages include those with conditions that cause abnormal drug distribution from the GI tract or from parenteral sites to the sites of action. Premature infants and patients with low serum protein levels or severe liver or kidney disease who can't metabolize or excrete drugs as readily as normal patients also require special drug dosages. You can help individualize drug regimens for these patients by assessing their kidney or liver function, monitoring blood levels or drugs, and calculating exact dosages.

Use correct units of measure

Using the incorrect unit of measure is one of the most common dosage errors. When calculating doses, matching units of measure in the numerator and denominator cancel each other, leaving the correct unit of measure in the answer. Here's an example:

How many milligrams of a drug are in two tablets if one tablet contains 5 mg of the drug?

☞ State the problem as a proportion:

$$5 \text{ mg} : 1 \text{ tablet} :: X \text{ mg} : 2 \text{ tablets}$$

✌ Remember that the product of the means equals the product of the extremes:

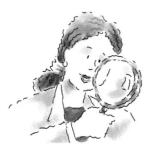

Multiply the means.

$$1 \text{ tablet} \times X \text{ mg} = 5 \text{ mg} \times 2 \text{ tablets}$$

Multiply the extremes.

☞ Solve for *X*. Divide each side of the equation by the known value, 1 tablet, and cancel units that appear in both the numerator and denominator:

$$\frac{1 \text{ tablet} \times X \text{ mg}}{1 \text{ tablet}} = \frac{5 \text{ mg} \times 2 \text{ tablets}}{1 \text{ tablet}}$$

$$X = 10 \text{ mg}$$

Double-check decimals and zeros

An error in the number of decimal places or zeros in a dosage calculation can cause a tenfold or greater dosage error. Here's an example using both decimals and zeros: The doctor orders *0.05 mg of Synthroid P.O.,* but the only Synthroid on hand is in tablet form, containing 0.025 mg each. How many tablets should you give?

☞ State the problem as a proportion:

$$0.025 \text{ mg} : 1 \text{ tablet} :: 0.05 \text{ mg} : X \text{ tablet}$$

✌ The product of the means equals the product of the extremes:

$$1 \text{ tablet} \times 0.05 \text{ mg} = 0.025 \text{ mg} \times X \text{ tablet}$$

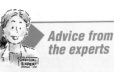

Advice from the experts

Helpful hints to minimize math mistakes

Avoid math mistakes when computing doses. Take a hint and use these helpful hints:

• First calculate the approximate dose in your head.
• Write out all calculations, using the proper formula.
• Recheck your calculations with another nurse or the pharmacist.

Solve for X. Divide each side of the equation by 0.025 mg and cancel units that appear in both the numerator and denominator, carefully checking decimal placement:

$$\frac{1 \text{ tablet} \times 0.05 \text{ mg}}{0.025 \text{ mg}} = \frac{0.025 \text{ mg} \times X \text{ tablet}}{0.025 \text{ mg}}$$

$$X = 2 \text{ tablets}$$

Question the answer

Be especially careful to recheck suspicious-looking calculations. For example, if a dosage calculation suggests giving 25 tablets or 200 ml of suspension, assume that you've made an error and recheck your figures. If you're still unsure about your results, have another nurse check your calculation.

Get out the calculator

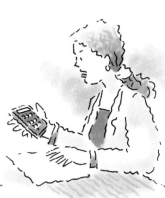

A handheld calculator can improve the accuracy and speed of your calculations, *but it can't guarantee accuracy.* You still must set up proportions carefully and double-check units of measure and decimal places.

Special considerations

Occasionally when administering oral drugs, you may come across unusual situations that require you to take a few extra steps.

Ticket to divide

Most tablets, capsules, and similar dosage forms are available in a few strengths only. Usually, you'll administer one tablet or one-half of a scored tablet.

Breaking an unscored tablet in portions smaller than one-half usually creates an inaccurate dose. If a dose smaller than one-half of a scored tablet or any portion of an unscored tablet is needed, you should substitute a commercially available solution or suspension or have one prepared by the pharmacist.

You can also ask the pharmacist to crush the tablet and weigh the exact dose. *However, some oral preparations shouldn't be opened, broken, scored, or crushed because this changes the drug's action.* (See *Take caution with tablets and capsules.*)

All things being equianalgesic

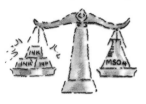

At times, you may need to convert a dose of an analgesic from the parenteral route to the oral route. If so, equianalgesic charts provide the information you need to recalculate the dose necessary to produce the desired pain control. These charts use morphine sulfate as the gold

Before you give that drug

Take caution with tablets and capsules

Before you break or crush a tablet or capsule, check your drug handbook to see if this will affect the drug's action. Drugs that shouldn't be altered include the following:
• sustained-release drugs, also called extended-release, timed-release, or controlled-release
• capsules that contain tiny beads of medication, although you may empty the contents of some capsules into a beverage, pudding, or applesauce
• enteric-coated tablets, which have a hard coating — usually shiny or glossy — that's designed to protect the upper GI tract from irritation
• buccal and sublingual tablets.

Tips for crushing and breaking
If you need to crush a tablet, use a chewable form, which is softer. The easiest method is to crush the tablet while it's still in its package, using a hemostat or pill crusher. You can also crush it with a mortar and pestle.

If you need to break a tablet, use one that's scored. Carefully cut the tablet on the score line with a scalpel or sterile needle. If you need to break an unscored tablet, have the pharmacist crush, weigh, and dispense it in two equal doses.

Also enlist the pharmacist's help when you need to break a tablet into smaller pieces than the score allows or when you must administer a portion of a capsule. But first, call to see if smaller doses are available, or if the drug comes in liquid form if your patient has trouble swallowing.

standard for comparing pain control. (See *Equianalgesic charts: A painless path for converting dosages*.)

Real world problems

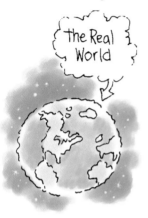

When calculating the number of tablets to administer, use proportions. Set up the first ratio or fraction with the known tablet strength. Set up the second ratio or fraction with the prescribed dose and the unknown quantity of tablets or capsules. Then solve for X to determine the correct dose. To illustrate, here are some typical patient situations.

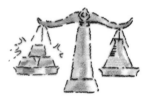

Equianalgesic charts: A painless path for converting dosages

When substituting one analgesic for another, equianalgesic charts provide the information you need to calculate the dose necessary to produce the desired pain control (equianalgesic effect).

These charts use morphine sulfate as the *gold standard* for comparison. On most charts, doses for a variety of drugs are listed; each dose provides pain relief equivalent to 10 mg of I.M. morphine. Here's an example of an equianalgesic chart:

Narcotic drugs: Equianalgesic doses

Medication	I.M. dose	P.O. dose
Morphine	10 mg	30 mg
Codeine	130 mg	200 mg
Hydromorphone	1.5 mg	7.5 mg
Levorphanol	2 mg	4 mg
Meperidine	75 mg	300 mg

Just remember: Every dose on the equianalgesic chart provides an equivalent amount of pain control.

The acetaminophen answer

The doctor orders *650 mg of acetaminophen* for your patient, but the drug is available only in 325-mg tablets. How many tablets should you give?

Here's the calculation using ratios:

• Set up the first ratio with the known tablet strength:

$$325 \text{ mg} : 1 \text{ tablet}$$

• Set up the second ratio with the desired dose and the unknown number of tablets:

$$650 \text{ mg} : X \text{ tablet}$$

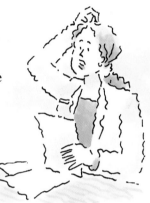

• Put these ratios into a proportion:

$$325 \text{ mg} : 1 \text{ tablet} :: 650 \text{ mg} : X \text{ tablet}$$

• Set up the equation by multiplying the means and the extremes:

$$1 \text{ tablet} \times 650 \text{ mg} = 325 \text{ mg} \times X \text{ tablet}$$

• Solve for X by dividing both sides of the equation by 325 mg and canceling units that appear in both the numerator and denominator:

$$\frac{1 \text{ tablet} \times 650 \,\cancel{\text{mg}}}{325 \,\cancel{\text{mg}}} = \frac{\cancel{325 \text{ mg}} \times X \text{ tablets}}{\cancel{325 \text{ mg}}}$$

$$X = 2 \text{ tablets}$$

The clozapine clue

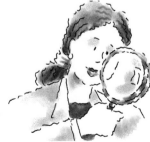

Your patient is prescribed 250 mg of clozapine P.O. daily. How many tablets should he take if each tablet is 100 mg?

Here's the calculation using ratios:

• Set up the first ratio with the known tablet strength:

$$100 \text{ mg} : 1 \text{ tablet}$$

• Set up the second ratio with the desired dose and the unknown number of tablets:

$$250 \text{ mg} : X \text{ tablet}$$

• Put these ratios into a proportion:

100 mg : 1 tablet :: 250 mg : X tablet

• Multiply the means and the extremes:

1 tablet × 250 mg = 100 mg × X tablet

• Divide each side of the equation by 100 mg and cancel units that appear in both the numerator and denominator:

$$\frac{1 \text{ tablet} \times 250 \text{ mg}}{100 \text{ mg}} = \frac{100 \text{ mg} \times X \text{ tablets}}{100 \text{ mg}}$$

$$X = 2\frac{1}{2} \text{ tablets}$$

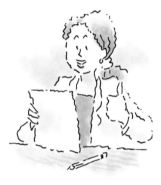

Enjoy the glyburide

The doctor's order reads *glyburide 1.5 mg iii tablets P.O. daily.* What is the total dose in milligrams?

Here's the solution using fractions:

• Set up the first fraction with the known tablet strength:

$$\frac{1.5 \text{ mg}}{1 \text{ tablet}}$$

• Set up the second fraction with the desired dose and the unknown number of milligrams:

$$\frac{X \text{ mg}}{3 \text{ tablets}}$$

• Put these fractions into a proportion:

$$\frac{X \text{ mg}}{3 \text{ tablets}} = \frac{1.5 \text{ mg}}{1 \text{ tablet}}$$

• Cross-multiply the fractions:

X mg × 1 tablet = 1.5 mg × 3 tablets

• Divide both sides of the equation by 1 tablet and cancel units that appear in both the numerator and denominator:

$$\frac{X \text{ mg} \times 1 \text{ tablet}}{1 \text{ tablet}} = \frac{3 \text{ tablets} \times 1.5 \text{ mg}}{1 \text{ tablet}}$$

$$X = 4.5 \text{ mg}$$

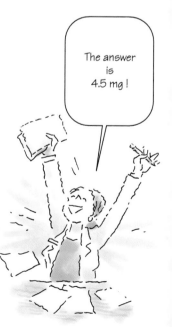

The answer is 4.5 mg!

Calculating liquid dosages

Besides administering tablets to your patients, you'll also give them liquid medications in suspension or elixir form. Before calculating a dose, read the label carefully to identify the dose strength in a specified amount of solution. Then check the label for the expiration date.

More real world problems

In the following problems, use the proportion method to calculate the amount of solution. Set up the first ratio or fraction with the known solution strength, and set up the second ratio or fraction with the desired dose and the unknown quantity. Then solve for X to find the correct dose.

Here are some typical patient situations.

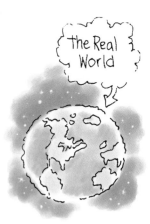

Pay attention to the suspension

Your patient is receiving 500 mg of Ceclor oral suspension. The label says Ceclor 250 mg/5 ml, and the bottle contains 100 ml. How many milliliters of Ceclor should you give?

Here's the solution, using fractions:

• Set up the first fraction with the known solution strength:

$$\frac{5 \text{ ml}}{250 \text{ mg}}$$

• Set up the second fraction with the desired dose and the unknown number of milliliters:

$$\frac{X \text{ ml}}{500 \text{ mg}}$$

• Put these fractions into a proportion:

$$\frac{X \text{ ml}}{500 \text{ mg}} = \frac{5 \text{ ml}}{250 \text{ mg}}$$

• Cross-multiply the fractions:

$$X \text{ ml} \times 250 \text{ mg} = 5 \text{ ml} \times 500 \text{ mg}$$

• Solve for X by dividing both sides of the equation by 250 mg and canceling units that appear in both the numerator and denominator:

$$\frac{X\,\text{ml} \times 250\,\text{mg}}{250\,\text{mg}} = \frac{5\,\text{ml} \times 500\,\text{mg}}{250\,\text{mg}}$$

$$X = \frac{2{,}500\,\text{ml}}{250}$$

$$X = 10\,\text{ml}$$

Erythromycin enigma

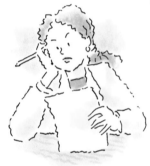

Your patient needs 400 mg of erythromycin oral suspension. The label says erythromycin 200 mg/5 ml. How many milliliters should you give?

Here's the calculation using ratios:

• Set up the first ratio with the known solution strength:

$$X\,\text{ml} : 400\,\text{mg}$$

• Set up the second ratio with the desired dose and the unknown number of milliliters:

$$5\,\text{ml} : 200\,\text{mg}$$

• Put these ratios into a proportion:

$$X\,\text{ml} : 400\,\text{mg} :: 5\,\text{ml} : 200\,\text{mg}$$

• Set up an equation by multiplying the extremes and the means:

$$X\,\text{ml} \times 200\,\text{mg} = 5\,\text{ml} \times 400\,\text{mg}$$

• Solve for X by dividing both sides of the equation by 200 mg and canceling units that appear in both the numerator and denominator:

$$\frac{X\,\text{ml} \times 200\,\text{mg}}{200\,\text{mg}} = \frac{5\,\text{ml} \times 400\,\text{mg}}{200\,\text{mg}}$$

$$X = \frac{2{,}000\,\text{ml}}{200}$$

$$X = 10\,\text{ml}$$

Don't dally over Dilantin doses

The doctor orders *100 mg of Dilantin oral suspension t.i.d.* for your patient. The label says Dilantin 125 mg/5 ml. How many milliliters should you give?

Here's the calculation using ratios:

• Set up the first fraction with the known solution strength:

$$X \text{ ml} : 100 \text{ mg}$$

• Set up the second fraction with the desired dose and the unknown number of milligrams:

$$5 \text{ ml} : 125 \text{ mg}$$

• Put these fractions into a proportion:

$$X \text{ ml} : 100 \text{ mg} :: 5 \text{ ml} : 125 \text{ mg}$$

• Set up an equation by multiplying the means and the extremes:

$$100 \text{ mg} \times 5 \text{ ml} = 125 \text{ mg} \times X \text{ ml}$$

• Solve for X by dividing each side of the equation by 125 mg and canceling units that appear in both the numerator and denominator:

$$\frac{100 \text{ mg} \times 5 \text{ ml}}{125 \text{ mg}} = \frac{125 \text{ mg} \times X \text{ ml}}{125 \text{ mg}}$$

$$\frac{500 \text{ ml}}{125} = X$$

$$X = 4 \text{ ml}$$

Diluting powders

Some drugs become unstable when they're stored as liquids, so they're supplied in powder form. Before giving these drugs, dilute them with the appropriate diluent, usually tap water. Read the drug label carefully to see how much diluent to add.

After adding the diluent, read the label again to determine the dose strength contained in the volume of fluid.

To calculate the dosage, use the ratio and proportion method.

Where's the weight? In the volume

The dose concentration in oral solutions is expressed as the weight — or dose strength — of the drug contained in a volume of solution. For example, Lasix oral solution is provided as 10 mg/ml. So the solution contains 10 mg of Lasix (drug weight) in 1 ml (solution volume).

Measuring oral solutions

To administer an oral solution accurately, measure it with a medicine cup, dropper, or syringe. Medicine cups are calibrated to measure solutions in milliliters, tablespoons, teaspoons, drams, and ounces. For accuracy, hold the cup at eye level while pouring the solution.

For good measure

Drugs that are prescribed in drops usually are packaged with a dropper. If not, use a standard dropper instead. They can be used to measure solutions in milliliters or teaspoons. After measuring and administering a drug from a multiple-dose container, store it as directed on the drug label.

Don't use syringes to give oral drugs — if you leave the tip on by mistake, the patient can swallow or aspirate it.

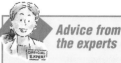

Advice from the experts

When you need a new measure

To easily determine a dose when you must first convert to a different system of measurement, remember these tips:
• Read the drug order thoroughly, paying close attention to decimal places and zeros.
• Convert the dose from the system in which it's ordered to the system in which it's available.
• Calculate the number of capsules or tablets or the amount of solution needed to obtain the desired dose.

Two-step dosage calculations

Most dosage calculations require more than one equation. For example, the doctor may order a drug in grains, but it may be available only in tablet, capsule, or liquid form in milligrams. When this happens, you need to convert from one measurement system to another before deciding how much medication to administer. (See *When you need a new measure.*)

Switch-hitting

When converting between measurement systems, first consult a conversion table to find the standard equivalent value — the equivalent between the two measurement systems. Then use the ratio and proportion method to calculate the correct dosage. Put the standard equivalent values in the first ratio or fraction, and put the quantity ordered and the unknown quantity in the second ratio or fraction.

Still more real world problems

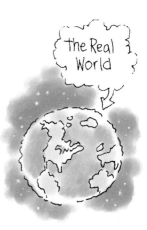

The Real World

The examples below show how to convert from one measurement system to another and then how to calculate the correct dose.

Be wary of the apothecary

Your patient's order, written in apothecaries' units, reads *aspirin gr x P.O.,* but the unit-dose package says aspirin 325 mg. How many tablets should you give?

Here's how to solve this using fractions:

• Recall that in apothecaries' units, "aspirin gr x" indicates 10 grains of aspirin. In this case, refer to *Measure for measure* on page 91, to find that 1 grain is equivalent to approximately 60 mg. Then set up the first fraction with the standard equivalent values:

$$\frac{60 \text{ mg}}{1 \text{ grain}}$$

• Set up the second fraction with the unknown quantity in the appropriate position:

$$\frac{X \text{ mg}}{10 \text{ grains}}$$

• Put these fractions into a proportion:

$$\frac{60 \text{ mg}}{1 \text{ grain}} = \frac{X \text{ mg}}{10 \text{ grains}}$$

• Cross-multiply the fractions to set up an equation:

$$60 \text{ mg} \times 10 \text{ grains} = X \text{ mg} \times 1 \text{ grain}$$

• Solve for *X* by dividing both sides of the equation by 1 grain and canceling units that appear in both the numerator and denominator:

$$\frac{60 \text{ mg} \times 10 \text{ grains}}{1 \text{ grain}} = \frac{X \text{ mg} \times 1 \text{ grain}}{1 \text{ grain}}$$

$$X = 600 \text{ mg}$$

• The dose to be given is 600 mg. Now determine the number of tablets to give by setting up a proportion:

$$\frac{X \text{ tablet}}{600 \text{ mg}} = \frac{1 \text{ tablet}}{325 \text{ mg}}$$

• Cross-multiply the fractions:

$$X \text{ tablet} \times 325 \text{ mg} = 1 \text{ tablet} \times 600 \text{ mg}$$

• Solve for X by dividing each side of the equation by 325 mg and canceling units that appear in both the numerator and denominator:

$$\frac{X \text{ tablets} \times 325 \text{ mg}}{325 \text{ mg}} = \frac{1 \text{ tablet} \times 600 \text{ mg}}{325 \text{ mg}}$$

$$X = \frac{600 \text{ tablets}}{325}$$

$$X = 1\tfrac{4}{5} \text{ tablets}$$

• Because giving 1⅘ tablets would be very difficult, round off the dose to 2 tablets.

Pondering a prescription

A prescription reads phenobarbital gr ¼; take gr ½ t.i.d. P.O. daily. How many milligrams of phenobarbital should this patient receive?

Here's how to solve this using fractions:
• Convert "gr ¼" to milligrams by consulting a conversion table such as the one in *Measure for measure* on page 91. You'll see that 1 grain equals approximately 60 mg.

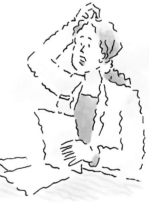

• Set up the first fraction with the standard equivalent values:

$$\frac{60 \text{ mg}}{1 \text{ grain}}$$

• Set up the second fraction with the unknown quantity in the appropriate position:

$$\frac{X \text{ mg}}{\text{grain } \frac{1}{4}}$$

• Put these fractions into an equation:

$$\frac{60 \text{ mg}}{1 \text{ grain}} = \frac{X \text{ mg}}{\text{grain } \frac{1}{4}}$$

• Cross-multiply the fractions:

$$60 \text{ mg} \times \text{grain } \tfrac{1}{4} = X \text{ mg} \times 1 \text{ grain}$$

• Solve for X by dividing each side of the equation by 1 grain and canceling units that appear in both the numerator and denominator:

$$\frac{X \text{ mg} \times 1 \cancel{\text{grain}}}{1 \cancel{\text{grain}}} = \frac{60 \text{ mg} \times \cancel{\text{grain}} \, \frac{1}{4}}{1 \cancel{\text{grain}}}$$

$$X = 60 \text{ mg} \times \tfrac{1}{4}$$

$$X = 15 \text{ mg}$$

• Now we know that grain $\frac{1}{4}$ equals 15 milligrams. However, the prescribed dose is grain $\frac{1}{2}$. Calculate the number of milligrams to give the patient by setting up a proportion:

$$\frac{X \text{ mg}}{\text{grain } \frac{1}{2}} = \frac{15 \text{ mg}}{\text{grain } \frac{1}{4}}$$

• Cross-multiply the fractions:

$$X \text{ mg} \times \text{grain } \tfrac{1}{4} = 15 \text{ mg} \times \text{grain } \tfrac{1}{2}$$

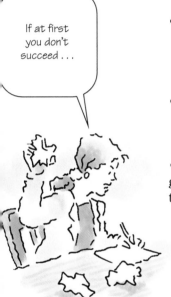

If at first you don't succeed . . .

• Solve for X by dividing both sides of the equation by grain ¼ and canceling units that appear in both the numerator and denominator:

$$\frac{X \text{ mg} \times \cancel{\text{grain } ¼}}{\cancel{\text{grain } ¼}} = \frac{15 \text{ mg} \times \cancel{\text{grain } ½}}{\cancel{\text{grain } ¼}}$$

$$X = \frac{15 \text{ mg} \times ½}{¼}$$

$$X = \frac{7½ \text{ mg}}{¼}$$

$$X = 30 \text{ mg}$$

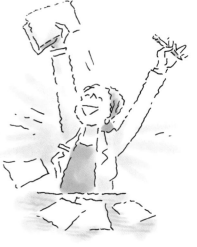

The dose to be given is 30 mg.

Digoxin diversion

Your patient receives a prescription for 62.5 mcg of digoxin elixir P.O. The elixir label reads 0.05 mg/ml. How many milliliters of digoxin should you give?

Here's how to solve this using ratios:

• Convert micrograms to milligrams. Recall that 1,000 mcg equals 1 mg.

• Set up the first ratio with this standard equivalent value:

$$1 \text{ mg} : 1,000 \text{ mcg}$$

• Set up the second ratio with the unknown quantity in the appropriate position:

$$X \text{ mg} : 62.5 \text{ mcg}$$

• Put these ratios into a proportion:

$$1 \text{ mg} : 1,000 \text{ mcg} :: X \text{ mg} : 62.5 \text{ mcg}$$

• Multiply the means and the extremes:

$$X \text{ mg} \times 1,000 \text{ mcg} = 1 \text{ mg} \times 62.5 \text{ mcg}$$

I knew
I should have paid
more attention in
math class!!!

• Solve for X by dividing both sides of the equation by 1,000 mcg and canceling units that appear in both the numerator and denominator:

$$\frac{X \text{ mg} \times 1{,}000 \text{ mcg}}{1{,}000 \text{ mcg}} = \frac{1 \text{ mg} \times 62.5 \text{ mcg}}{1{,}000 \text{ mcg}}$$

$$X = \frac{62.5 \text{ mg}}{1{,}000}$$

$$X = 0.0625 \text{ mg}$$

• The prescribed dose is 62.5 mcg, or 0.0625 mg. Calculate the number of milliliters to be given by setting up a proportion:

$$0.0625 \text{ mg} : X \text{ ml} :: 0.05 \text{ mg} : 1 \text{ ml}$$

• Set up an equation by multiplying the means and the extremes:

$$X \text{ ml} \times 0.05 \text{ mg} = 1 \text{ ml} \times 0.0625 \text{ mg}$$

• Solve for X by dividing each side of the equation by 0.05 mg and canceling the units of measure that appear in both the numerator and denominator:

$$\frac{X \text{ ml} \times 0.05 \text{ mg}}{0.05 \text{ mg}} = \frac{1 \text{ ml} \times 0.0625 \text{ mg}}{0.05 \text{ mg}}$$

$$X = 1.25 \text{ ml}$$

The dose to be given is 1.25 ml.

The desired-over-have method

The desired-over-have method is another way to solve two-step problems. This method uses fractions to express the known and unknown quantities in proportions:

$$\frac{\text{amount desired}}{\text{amount you have}} = \frac{\text{equivalent amount desired}}{\text{equivalent amount you have}}$$

Make sure the units of measure used in the numerator and denominator of the first fraction correspond to the units of measure in the numerator and denominator of the second fraction.

Three examples (count 'em)

The following three problems show how to use the desired-over-have method.

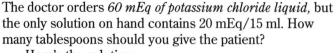

The potassium chloride puzzler

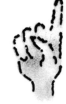

The doctor orders *60 mEq of potassium chloride liquid,* but the only solution on hand contains 20 mEq/15 ml. How many tablespoons should you give the patient?

Here's the solution:

• Convert milliliters to tablespoons by consulting a conversion table such as the one in *Measure for measure* on page 91. You'll see that 15 ml equals 1 tbs. Therefore, 20 mEq of the solution on hand equals 1 tbs.

• Set up the first fraction with the amount desired over the amount you have:

$$\frac{60 \text{ mEq}}{20 \text{ mEq}}$$

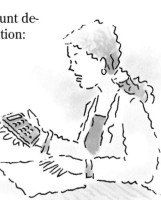

• Set up the second fraction with the unknown amount desired — represented by X — in the appropriate position:

$$\frac{X \text{ tbs}}{1 \text{ tbs}}$$

• Put these fractions into a proportion:

$$\frac{X \text{ tbs desired}}{1 \text{ tbs have}} = \frac{60 \text{ mEq desired}}{20 \text{ mEq have}}$$

• Cross-multiply the fractions:

$$X \text{ tbs} \times 20 \text{ mEq} = 1 \text{ tbs} \times 60 \text{ mEq}$$

• Solve for X by dividing each side of the equation by 20 mEq and canceling units that appear in both the numerator and denominator:

$$\frac{X \text{ tbs} \times 20 \text{ mEq}}{20 \text{ mEq}} = \frac{1 \text{ tbs} \times 60 \text{ mEq}}{20 \text{ mEq}}$$

$$X = 3 \text{ tbs}$$

The patient should receive 3 tbs of potassium chloride liquid.

Acetaminophen alley

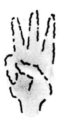

The order reads *acetaminophen elixir 650 mg P.O. stat.* The pharmacy sends you Tylenol 325 mg/5 ml. How many teaspoons do you give?

Here's the calculation:

• Convert milliliters to teaspoons by consulting a conversion table such as the one in *Measure for measure* on page 91. You'll see that 1 tsp equals 5 ml.

• Set up the first fraction with the amount desired over the amount you have:

$$\frac{650 \text{ mg}}{325 \text{ mg}}$$

• Set up the second fraction with the unknown amount desired in the appropriate position:

$$\frac{X \text{ tsp}}{1 \text{ tsp}}$$

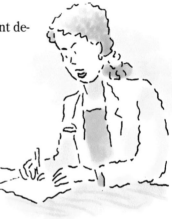

• Put these fractions into a proportion:

$$\frac{X \text{ tsp desired}}{1 \text{ tsp have}} = \frac{650 \text{ mg desired}}{325 \text{ mg have}}$$

• Cross-multiply the fractions:

$$X \text{ tsp} \times 325 \text{ mg} = 1 \text{ tsp} \times 650 \text{ mg}$$

• Solve for *X* by dividing both sides of the equation by 325 mg and canceling units that appear in both the numerator and denominator:

$$\frac{X \text{ tsp} \times \cancel{325 \text{ mg}}}{\cancel{325 \text{ mg}}} = \frac{1 \text{ tsp} \times 650 \cancel{\text{ mg}}}{325 \cancel{\text{ mg}}}$$

$$X = 2 \text{ tsp}$$

The patient should receive 2 tsp of acetaminophen elixir.

Teaspoon teaser

The doctor orders *60 mg of phenobarbital elixir* for your patient, but the drug is only available as 20 mg/5 ml. How many teaspoons should you give?

Here's the calculation:
• Convert milliliters to teaspoons by consulting a conversion chart. You'll see that 1 tsp equals 5 ml.
• Set up the first fraction with the amount desired over the amount you have:

$$\frac{60 \text{ mg}}{20 \text{ mg}}$$

• Set up the second fraction with the unknown amount desired in the appropriate position:

$$\frac{X \text{ tsp}}{1 \text{ tsp}}$$

• Put these fractions into a proportion:

$$\frac{60 \text{ mg}}{20 \text{ mg}} = \frac{X \text{ tsp}}{1 \text{ tsp}}$$

• Cross-multiply the fractions:

$$60 \text{ mg} \times 1 \text{ tsp} = 20 \text{ mg} \times X \text{ tsp}$$

• Solve for X by dividing both sides of the equation by 20 mg and canceling units that appear in both the numerator and denominator:

$$\frac{60 \text{ mg} \times 1 \text{ tsp}}{20 \text{ mg}} = \frac{20 \text{ mg} \times X \text{ tsp}}{20 \text{ mg}}$$

$$\frac{60 \text{ tsp}}{20} = X$$

$$3 \text{ tsp} = X$$

You should give the patient 3 tsp of phenobarbital elixir.

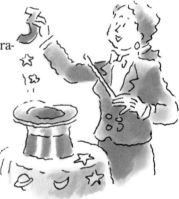

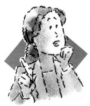

Quick quiz

1. One tablet of Lasix contains 40 mg, so three tablets contain:
   A. 120 mg
   B. 150 mg
   C. 180 mg

Answer: A. If each tablet is 40 mg, multiply 40 by 3 to find the answer: 120 mg.

2. If a patient needs 100 mcg of Synthroid P.O., and the available dose is 25 mcg/tablet, the number of tablets to give is:

    A. 4
    B. 6
    C. 7

Answer: A. If 1 tablet provides 25 mcg, divide 100 by 25 to get the answer: 4 tablets.

3. If 250 mg of Clozaril is ordered for a patient, but only 100-mg tablets are available, you should give:

    A. 2 tablets.
    B. 2½ tablets.
    C. 3½ tablets.

Answer: B. By dividing 250 by 100, you get 2.5, or 2½ tablets.

4. When reading a drug label, first check the:

    A. dose strength.
    B. generic name.
    C. trade name.

Answer: B. The generic name follows the trade name on a drug label.

5. If the doctor orders *640 mg of Tylenol liquid,* and the bottle label says Tylenol 80 mg/½ teaspoon, you should give the patient:

    A. 15 ml
    B. 20 ml
    C. 25 ml

Answer: B. First, consult a conversion table to find that 1 tsp equals 5 ml. Then use proportions to solve for X.

6. If 80 mg of Lasix oral solution is ordered, and Lasix 10 mg/ml is available, you should administer:

    A. 8 ml
    B. 10 ml
    C. 12 ml

Answer: A. Use proportions to solve for X.

7. If a dose smaller than one-half of a scored tablet is needed, you should:

    A. substitute a commercially available solution or suspension or one prepared by the pharmacist.

    B. cut the tablet with a knife.

    C. break the tablet with your hand.

Answer: A. Breaking an unscored tablet in portions smaller than one-half usually yields an incorrect dose.

Scoring

☆☆☆   If you answered all seven items correctly, excellent! Expressed as a ratio it's 7 : 7 :: 100 : 100 (in other words, perfect).

☆☆   If you answered five or six correctly, good job! Your calculation skills are stupendous (but, remember, a good calculator never hurt anybody).

☆   If you answered fewer than five correctly, don't worry! Keep on calculatin' (whether it's milligrams or milliliters).

Calculating topical and rectal drug dosages

Just the facts

In this chapter, you'll learn:

♦ how to interpret topical and rectal drug labels

♦ what types of drugs are given topically and rectally and how they work

♦ how to perform dosage calculations for topical and rectal drugs.

A look at topical and rectal drugs

Some types of drugs must be administered by the topical, or dermal, route. These drugs include creams, lotions, ointments, and powders, which commonly are used for dermatologic treatment or wound care, or patches, which have various uses, including treating angina. Topical drugs are applied to the skin and absorbed through the epidermis into the dermis.

Drugs also may be given rectally. This route may be preferred for patients who can't take drugs orally, such as those with nasogastric tubes, nausea, or vomiting. It also may be used with unconscious patients who can't swallow, and to achieve specific local and systemic effects. Rectal drugs include enemas and suppositories.

The label says it

Three rules for administering medication: Read the label, read the label, read the label.

A topical topic

When reading a topical ointment label, note the following information as shown on the box label below:

- trade name (Bactroban)
- generic name (mupirocin)
- dose strength (2% ointment)
- total package volume (15 grams)
- special instructions (not included on this label).

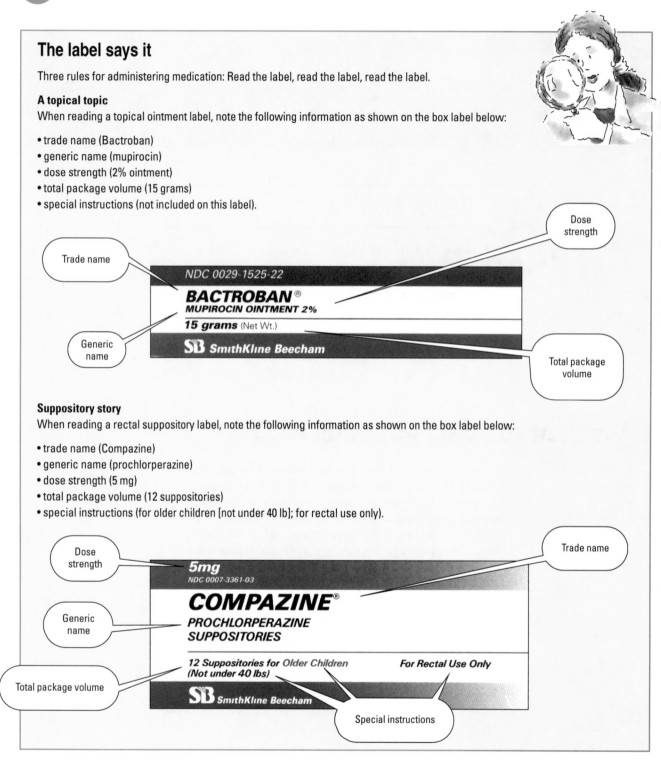

Dose strength

Trade name

NDC 0029-1525-22

BACTROBAN®
MUPIROCIN OINTMENT 2%

15 grams (Net Wt.)

SB SmithKline Beecham

Generic name

Total package volume

Suppository story

When reading a rectal suppository label, note the following information as shown on the box label below:

- trade name (Compazine)
- generic name (prochlorperazine)
- dose strength (5 mg)
- total package volume (12 suppositories)
- special instructions (for older children [not under 40 lb]; for rectal use only).

Dose strength

Trade name

5mg
NDC 0007-3361-03

COMPAZINE®
PROCHLORPERAZINE SUPPOSITORIES

12 Suppositories for Older Children **(Not under 40 lbs)**   **For Rectal Use Only**

SB SmithKline Beecham

Generic name

Total package volume

Special instructions

Read the label

When you read the labels on topical and rectal drugs, look for the same information as you would with oral and parenteral drugs. (See *The label says it.*) The trade name appears first, followed by the generic name, the dose strength, and the total volume of the package. (See *Combination product alert.*) Labels also may contain special administration instructions. Sometimes, the print on the labels is quite small, so look carefully.

Transdermal patches

In the past, topical drugs were used almost solely for their local effects. But today, several transdermal drugs are used for their systemic effects as well.

I've got you under my skin

Transdermal patch drugs penetrate the outer layers of the skin by way of passive diffusion at a constant rate; then the drugs are absorbed into the circulation. Patches are a good way to administer drugs that aren't absorbed well in the GI tract, or those that are metabolized and eliminated too quickly to be effective.

Good news and bad news

Patches are convenient and easy to use, and they maintain consistent blood levels. However, they also have disadvantages. Their onset of action is slow, so a therapeutic blood level takes hours or even days to achieve. Patches also need to be checked frequently, especially if the patient is active, because they may become displaced. In addition, reversing toxic effects of patches can be difficult because the drug takes so long to metabolize.

Release me

Drug concentrations in transdermal patches vary depending on the design of the patch, but the concentration isn't as important as the drug's rate of release. Two patches containing the same drug in different concentrations may actually release the same amount of drug per hour.

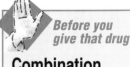

Before you give that drug

Combination product alert

Topical preparations may contain more than one drug. For example, Mycitracin Plus ointment contains bacitracin, neomycin, polymyxin B, and lidocaine. Carefully note all ingredients when checking labels, and be sure that your patient isn't allergic to any of them.

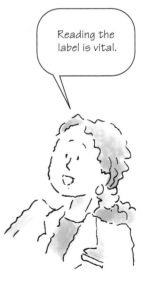

Reading the label is vital.

A batch of patches

Patches are available for a variety of conditions, including a nitroglycerin patch to prevent angina, a clonidine patch to control hypertension, and a fentanyl patch to manage chronic pain.

The fentanyl transdermal system, or Duragesic patch, is an example of a transdermal drug used systemically. It's held in a reservoir behind a membrane that allows controlled drug absorption through the skin. These patches are available in doses of 25, 50, 75, and 100 mcg/hour, with the higher doses used for opioid-resistant patients. To ensure that the patient receives the correct dose, change the patch every 72 hours, and check the label to verify the fentanyl dosage. (See *Prescribed patches.*)

Prescribed patches

The following transdermal drugs allow you to topically administer systemic drugs.

Nitroglycerin

Transdermal nitroglycerin provides prophylactic treatment of chronic angina. Available brands include Deponit, Nitrodisc, Nitro-Dur, and Transderm-Nitro. A new patch is applied daily (usually in the morning) and removed after 12 to 14 hours to prevent the patient from developing a tolerance to the drug.

Nicotine

This transdermal medication is used to treat smoking addiction. Brands include Habitrol, Nicoderm, Nicotrol, and ProStep. These drugs should be used only as an adjunct to a behavioral therapy program. A new patch is applied daily. Nicotrol should be removed after 16 hours, but other brands should stay on for 24 hours.

Clonidine

This drug is used to treat hypertension. The brand name for this drug is Catapres TTS. A new patch is applied every 7 days.

Fentanyl

Fentanyl is administered to treat severe chronic pain. Its brand name is Duragesic. Each patch may be worn up to 72 hours.

Scopolamine

Scopolamine is used to treat nausea, vomiting, and vertigo. Brands include Transderm-Scōp and Transderm-V (available in Canada). The patch is applied to skin behind the ear at least 4 hours before an antiemetic effect is needed. It can be worn for three days.

Estradiol

This transdermal drug provides hormonal replacement to estrogen deficient women. The brand names include Climara, Estraderm, and Vivelle. It's administered on an intermittent cyclic schedule (3 weeks of therapy followed by discontinuation for 1 week).

Testosterone

This transdermal drug provides hormonal replacement for men with testosterone deficiency. The brand names are Androderm and Testoderm. The Testoderm patch is applied once daily to clean, hairless scrotal skin, which is the only skin that's thin enough to allow adequate blood levels.

Topical drug dosages

Topical drug dosages require very little calculating. As discussed above, transdermal patches are changed at regular intervals to ensure that the patient receives the correct dose. To apply a patch, simply remove the old patch and replace it with a new one at the appropriate time, following the manufacturer's guidelines.

Up to you

When the doctor prescribes an ointment as part of wound care or dermatologic treatment, he usually leaves the amount to apply up to you. He may give general guidance, such as "use a thin layer" or "apply thickly." When an ointment contains a drug intended for a systemic effect, more specific administration guidelines are necessary.

Many ointments, including nitroglycerin, are available in tubes. To apply ointment from a tube, use a paper ruler applicator to measure the correct dose. (See *Measuring a topical dose,* page 162.)

Calculating rectal drug dosages

Rectal drugs include enemas and suppositories. Suppositories are the most common form of rectal drugs.

To calculate the number of suppositories to give, use the proportion method with ratios or fractions. The doctor usually prescribes drugs in the dose provided by one suppository, but occasionally you may need to insert two suppositories. (See *Check and check again.*)

Real world problems

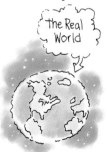

The Real World

The problems below illustrate how to calculate suppository dosages.

Your pediatric patient needs 240 mg of acetaminophen by suppository. The package label reads acetaminophen suppositories 120 mg. How many suppositories should you give?

Here's how to solve this problem using fractions:

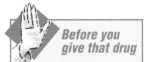

Before you give that drug

Check and check again

Occasionally you may need to insert more or less than one suppository. Here's what to do:

More than one

Do your dosage calculations indicate a need for more than one suppository? If so, check your figures and ask another nurse to check them, too. Then ask the pharmacist whether the suppository is available in other dose strengths.

More than two

If more than two suppositories are needed, confirm the dosage with the doctor. Then check with the pharmacist. He may be able to give you one suppository instead of multiple ones.

Less than one

If less than one suppository is needed, check your calculations and have another nurse do the same. Then ask the pharmacist if the dose is available in one suppository. This ensures the most accurate dose.

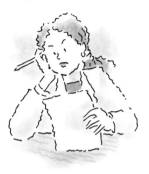

• Set up the first fraction with the known suppository dose:

$$\frac{1 \text{ supp}}{120 \text{ mg}}$$

• Set up the second fraction with the desired dose and the unknown number of suppositories:

$$\frac{X \text{ supp}}{240 \text{ mg}}$$

• Put these fractions into a proportion:

$$\frac{1 \text{ supp}}{120 \text{ mg}} = \frac{X \text{ supp}}{240 \text{ mg}}$$

• Cross-multiply the fractions:

$$120 \text{ mg} \times X \text{ supp} = 1 \text{ supp} \times 240 \text{ mg}$$

• Solve for X by dividing each side of the equation by 120 mg and canceling units that appear in both the numerator and denominator:

$$\frac{\cancel{120 \text{ mg}} \times X \text{ supp}}{\cancel{120 \text{ mg}}} = \frac{1 \text{ supp} \times 240 \cancel{\text{ mg}}}{120 \cancel{\text{ mg}}}$$

$$X = 2 \text{ suppositories}$$

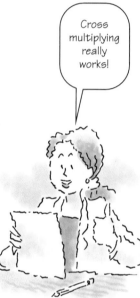

Cross multiplying really works!

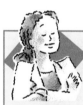

Peak technique

Measuring a topical dose

To measure a specified amount of ointment from a tube, squeeze the prescribed length of ointment in inches or centimeters onto a paper ruler like the one shown here. Then use the ruler to apply the ointment to the patient's skin at the appropriate time, following the manufacturer's guidelines for administration.

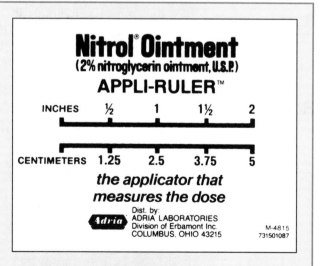

Nitrol® Ointment
(2% nitroglycerin ointment, U.S.P.)
APPLI-RULER™

| INCHES | ½ | 1 | 1½ | 2 |

| CENTIMETERS | 1.25 | 2.5 | 3.75 | 5 |

the applicator that measures the dose

Dist. by:
Adria ADRIA LABORATORIES
Division of Erbamont Inc.
COLUMBUS, OHIO 43215

M-4815
731501087

Example numero two

The doctor's order states *Dulcolax 10 mg per rectum at 6 a.m.* You only have 5-mg suppositories on hand. How many suppositories should you give this patient?

Here's how to solve this using fractions:
• Set up the first fraction with the known suppository dose:

$$\frac{1 \text{ supp}}{5 \text{ mg}}$$

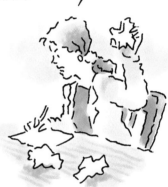

Say it
100 times . . .
I love math . . .
I love math . . .
I love math . . .

• Set up the second fraction with the desired dose and the unknown number of suppositories:

$$\frac{X \text{ supp}}{10 \text{ mg}}$$

• Put these fractions into a proportion:

$$\frac{1 \text{ supp}}{5 \text{ mg}} = \frac{X \text{ supp}}{10 \text{ mg}}$$

• Cross-multiply the fractions:

$$1 \text{ supp} \times 10 \text{ mg} = X \text{ supp} \times 5 \text{ mg}$$

• Solve for *X* by dividing each side of the equation by 5 mg and canceling units that appear in both the numerator and denominator:

$$\frac{1 \text{ supp} \times 10 \text{ mg}}{5 \text{ mg}} = \frac{X \text{ supp} \times 5 \text{ mg}}{5 \text{ mg}}$$

$$X = 2 \text{ suppositories}$$

Our last example: El grand finale

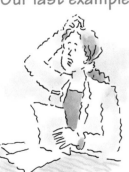

The doctor orders a *100-mg Tigan suppository* for your patient. The pharmacy is closed, and the only Tigan on hand contains 200 mg per suppository. How many suppositories should you give?

Here's how to solve this using ratios:
• Set up the first ratio with the known suppository dose:

$$1 \text{ supp} : 200 \text{ mg}$$

• Set up the second ratio with the desired dose and the unknown number of suppositories:

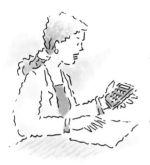

$$X \text{ supp} : 100 \text{ mg}$$

- Put these ratios into a proportion:

$$1 \text{ supp} : 200 \text{ mg} :: X \text{ supp} : 100 \text{ mg}$$

- Multiply the means and the extremes:

$$200 \text{ mg} \times X \text{ supp} = 100 \text{ mg} \times 1 \text{ supp}$$

- Solve for X by dividing each side of the equation by 200 mg and canceling units that appear in both the numerator and denominator:

$$\frac{200 \text{ mg} \times X \text{ supp}}{200 \text{ mg}} = \frac{100 \text{ mg} \times 1 \text{ supp}}{200 \text{ mg}}$$

$$X = \frac{1}{2} \text{ suppository}$$

YIPPEEE!
I'm finished
(at least until
the next
chapter).

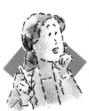

Quick quiz

1. According to the label below, the generic name of this drug is:

    A. Retin-A Gel.

    B. tretinoin.

    C. hydroxypropyl cellulose.

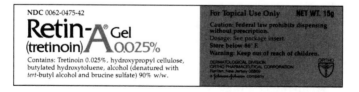

NDC 0062-0475-42

Retin-A Gel
(tretinoin) 0.025%

Contains: Tretinoin 0.025%, hydroxypropyl cellulose, butylated hydroxytoluene, alcohol (denatured with *tert*-butyl alcohol and brucine sulfate) 90% w/w.

For Topical Use Only   NET WT. 15g

Caution: Federal law prohibits dispensing without prescription.
Dosage: See package insert.
Store below 86° F.
Warning: Keep out of reach of children.

DERMATOLOGICAL DIVISION
ORTHO PHARMACEUTICAL CORPORATION
Raritan, New Jersey 08869
a Johnson-Johnson company

Answer: B. On drug labels, the generic name always appears after the trade name.

2. Transdermal patches used to relieve chronic pain are effective for many hours due to:
  A. controlled absorption through the skin.
  B. enhanced effect on local tissue.
  C. rapid then slow release of analgesics.

Answer: A. These drugs are slowly released and absorbed through the skin over a period of time.

3. A commonly used transdermal drug is:
  A. Scoline.
  B. nitroglycerin.
  C. M S Contin.

Answer: B. Nitroglycerin patches are used to prevent angina.

4. If a drug label reads *Compazine (prochlorperazine) suppositories 5 mg, SmithKline Beecham, for rectal use only,* the drug's proprietary name is:
  A. Compazine.
  B. prochlorperazine.
  C. SmithKline Beecham.

Answer: A. The proprietary or trade name always appears first on a drug label.

5. If the doctor's order reads *Nitrol Ointment 1″ q6h,* you should measure this dose:
  A. on a paper ruler applicator.
  B. by using your own judgment to approximate 1″ of ointment.
  C. by holding a wooden ruler to the patient's skin to measure the ointment.

Answer: A. Nitrol Ointment comes with its own paper ruler. Squeeze the prescribed length of ointment onto the ruler, and then use the ruler to apply the ointment to the patient's skin.

6. If a patient needs 500 mg of aminophylline by suppository, but all you have are 250-mg suppositories, you should insert:
  A. 1 suppository.
  B. 2 suppositories.
  C. 3 suppositories.

Answer: B. A simple calculation tells you that the patient needs 2 suppositories. However, because more than 1 suppository is needed, you should check your calculations, have another nurse do the same, and then call the pharmacy to see if a 500-mg dose is available.

7. When a doctor prescribes antibiotic ointment for a finger laceration, you should:

    A. ask him to prescribe a specific amount.

    B. use a paper applicator to apply the ointment.

    C. use your own judgment about the amount of ointment to apply.

Answer: C. Unless the ointment has a systemic effect, the doctor will usually leave the amount to apply up to you.

8. If a child needs 2.5 mg of Compazine, and the package label reads *Compazine suppositories 5 mg,* you should give:

    A. 2 suppositories.

    B. ½ suppository.

    C. 1 suppository.

Answer: B. By setting up a proportion and solving for *X,* you'll find that the child needs ½ of a 5-mg suppository.

Scoring

☆☆☆ If you answered all eight items correctly, wow! You know your routes better than AAA!

☆☆ If you answered five to seven correctly, all right! You'll soon be top dog in topical drug administration!

☆ If you answered fewer than five correctly, good job! You're absorbing information at an incredible rate!

Part V

Parenteral administration

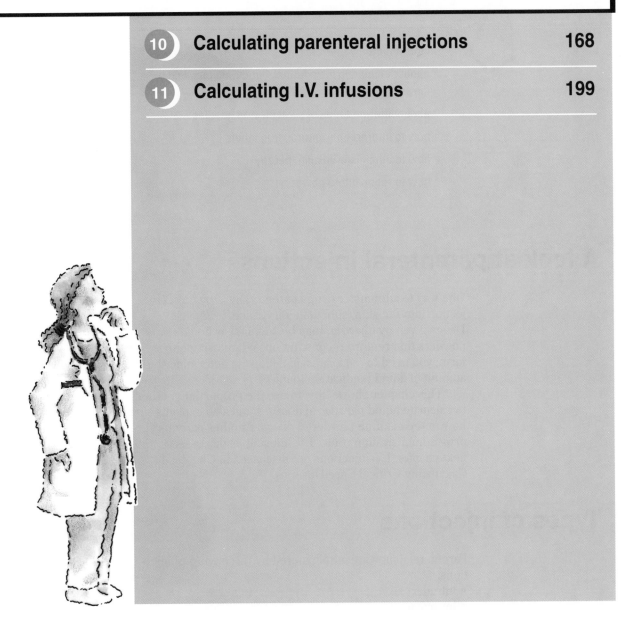

Calculating parenteral injections

Just the facts

In this chapter, you'll learn:

♦ about calculating intradermal, subcutaneous, and intramuscular injections

♦ about different types of syringes and needles

♦ how to interpret parenteral drug labels

♦ how to administer insulin therapy

♦ how to reconstitute powders.

A look at parenteral injections

One way to administer drugs parenterally is by direct injection into the skin, subcutaneous tissue, or muscle. Drugs given by injection may be supplied as liquids or as powders that require reconstitution. When using either form, you need to perform calculations to determine the amount of liquid medication to inject.

This chapter shows how to use the proportion method to calculate liquid parenteral dosages and also explains how to reconstitute powdered drugs. Another parenteral drug administration route, I.V. infusion, is discussed in the next chapter. I.V. injections are discussed in Chapter 14, Calculating Critical Care Dosages.

Types of injections

Parenteral drugs are administered by three types of injections:
• intradermal
• intravenous

- subcutaneous
- intramuscular.

Giving parenteral drugs safely depends on choosing the right type of injection for the patient's condition and the right syringe and needle for the type of injection.

Intradermal injections

In an intradermal injection, medication is injected into the dermis — the layer of skin beneath the epidermis, which is the outermost layer of skin. This type of injection is used to anesthetize the skin for invasive procedures and to test for allergies or tuberculosis, histoplasmosis, and other diseases.

I've got you intra my skin

The volume of a drug that's given by intradermal injection is less than 0.5 ml. A 1-ml syringe, calibrated in 0.01-ml increments, is usually used, along with a 26-to 27-gauge (G) needle that's ½″ to ⅝″ long.

To perform an intradermal injection, use the following basic procedure:
- Clean the skin thoroughly.
- Stretch the skin taut with one hand.
- With your other hand, insert the needle quickly at a 10- to 15-degree angle to a depth of about 0.5 cm.
- Inject the drug. A small wheal forms where the drug is injected into the skin.

Subcutaneous injections

In a subcutaneous (S.C.) injection, the drug is injected into the subcutaneous tissue, which is below the dermis and above the muscle. Drugs are absorbed faster in this layer than in the dermis because this layer has more capillaries. Insulin, heparin, tetanus toxoid, and some narcotics are injected through this route.

More than skin deep

Only 0.5 to 1.5 ml of a drug can be injected S.C. The needles used for S.C. injections are 25G to 27G and ½″ to ⅝″ long. S.C. injection sites include:
- the lateral areas of the upper arms and thighs
- the abdomen above, below, and lateral to the umbilicus
- the upper back.

To perform an S.C. injection, use the following basic procedure:

• Choose the injection site.
• Clean the skin.
• If the patient is thin, pinch the skin between your index finger and thumb, and insert the needle at a 45-degree angle.
• If the patient is obese, insert the needle into the fatty tissue at a 90-degree angle.
• Aspirate for blood (this isn't mandatory).
• Administer the injection.
• Massage the site after removing the needle; this may enhance absorption.

Intramuscular injections

An intramuscular (I.M.) injection, which goes into a muscle, is used for drugs that need to be absorbed quickly or that irritate the tissues. The volume for these injections ranges from 0.5 to 3 ml. I.M. injection sites include:

• the ventral gluteal or vastus lateralis muscle for 3-ml injections
• the rectus femoris or deltoid muscle for injections less than 3 ml.

The choice of injection site depends on the patient's muscle mass and overlying tissue and the volume of the injection.

Use a little muscle

To administer an I.M. injection, follow this basic procedure:

• Choose the injection site.
• Clean the skin.
• Using a quick, dartlike action, insert the needle at a 75- to 90-degree angle.
• Before injecting the drug, aspirate to make sure the needle isn't in a vein.
• Push the plunger and keep the syringe steady.
• After the drug is injected, pull the needle straight out and apply pressure to the site.

Syringes and needles

Several types of syringes and needles are used to administer parenteral drugs. Each syringe and needle is designed for a different purpose.

Types of syringes

To measure and administer parenteral drugs, three basic types of hypodermic syringes are used: standard syringes, tuberculin syringes, and prefilled syringes. Although these syringes are sometimes calibrated in cubic centimeters, the drugs they're used to measure are commonly ordered in milliliters. (Recall that 1 cc equals 1 ml and that milliliters and cubic centimeters are used interchangeably.)

Standard syringes

Standard syringes are available in 3, 5, 10, 20, 30, 50, and 60 ml. Each syringe consists of a plunger, a barrel, a hub, a needle, and dead space. (See *Anatomy of a syringe*.) The dead space holds fluid that remains in the syringe and needle after the plunger is completely depressed. Some syringes, such as insulin syringes, don't have dead space.

Anatomy of a syringe

Standard syringes come in many different sizes, but each syringe has the same components. The illustration below shows the parts of a standard syringe.

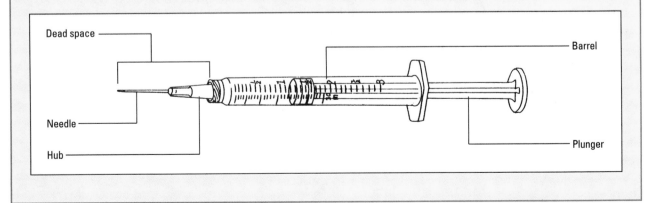

Dead space

Barrel

Needle

Hub

Plunger

Marked for good measure

The calibration marks on syringes allow you to accurately measure drug doses. The 3-ml syringe, which is the syringe that's most commonly used, is calibrated in tenths of a milliliter on the right and minims on the left. It has large marks for ½ ml on the right. The large-volume syringes are calibrated in 2- to 10-ml increments.

To administer a drug, follow these basic steps:
• Use aseptic technique.
• Calculate the dose.
• Draw the drug into the syringe.
• Pull the plunger back until the top ring of the plunger's black portion aligns with the correct calibration mark.
• Double check the dose measurement.
• Administer the drug.

Double the fun

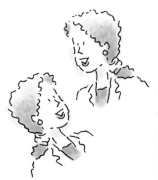

Parenteral drugs come in various dose strengths or concentrations so that the usual adult dose can be contained in 1 to 3 ml of solution. If a patient needs a dose larger than 3 ml, give it in two injections at two different sites to ensure proper drug absorption.

Tuberculin syringes

Tuberculin syringes are commonly used for intradermal injections and to administer small amounts of drugs, such as to pediatric patients or those on intensive care units. Each syringe is calibrated in hundredths of a milliliter on the right and minims on the left, allowing you to accurately administer doses as small as 0.25 ml. Tuberculin syringes are also marked for alternate tenths of a milliliter: 0.2, 0.4, 0.6, and 0.8 ml. (See *Touring a tuberculin syringe.*)

Measure drugs in a tuberculin syringe the same as you would with a standard syringe. But take extra care when reading the dose, because the measurements on the tuberculin syringe are very small.

Prefilled syringes

A sterile syringe filled with a premeasured dose of drug is called a prefilled syringe. These syringes usually come with a cartridge-needle unit and require a special holder called a Carpuject or Tubex to release the drug from the cartridge. Each cartridge is calibrated in tenths of a milliliter and has larger marks for half and full milliliters. (See *Previewing a prefilled syringe,* page 174.)

Room for one more

Some cartridges are designed so that a diluent or a second drug can be added when a combined dose is ordered. For example, many narcotics, such as meperidine (Demerol), come from the manufacturer in prefilled syringes. Because Demerol is often ordered along with hydroxyzine (Vistaril), the Demerol cartridge allows for the addition of Vistaril. *Always check a compatibility chart when mixing more than one drug in a single administration.*

First, the advantages...

Prefilled syringes have many advantages over multiple-dose vials. Because they're labeled with the drug name and dose, preparation time is reduced and so is the risk of drug errors.

This labeling also makes it easier to record the amount of drug used and eliminates the need to figure out how much drug is left in a vial after you've given an injection. This is especially important with narcotic doses, which the law says must be recorded exactly.

Touring a tuberculin syringe

A tuberculin syringe has the same components as a standard syringe. However, size and calibration of the syringe are distinct. Because the measurements on the tuberculin syringe are so small, take extra care when reading the dose.

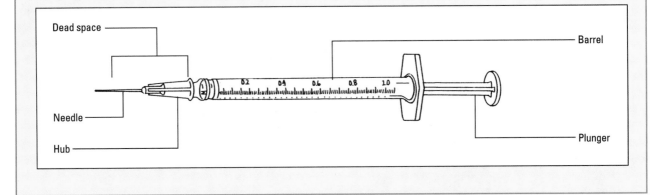

The most obvious advantage of prefilled syringes is that you don't have to measure each drug dose. The manufacturer has already done this and placed the dose in the syringe. *However, be aware that most manufacturers add a little extra drug to the syringe in case some is wasted when the syringe is purged of air.*

...Next, the disadvantages

Unfortunately, prefilled syringes aren't available in all possible doses. When the ordered dose doesn't match the amount in the prefilled syringe, you'll need to calculate the correct amount of drug needed.

After giving the injection, discard the extra drug by expelling it from the syringe. If the drug is a narcotic, document carefully the amount of drug you discard. Have another nurse witness the expulsion of the drug and then co-sign the narcotic record.

Closed-system devices

Another type of prefilled syringe, a closed-system device, comes with a needle and syringe in place and a separate prefilled drug chamber. Emergency drugs, such as at-

---

Previewing a prefilled syringe

The illustration below shows the parts of a prefilled syringe. Take note of the holder at right. The most commonly used brands of prefilled syringes are Carpuject and Tubex.

Drug label

Dead space

Cartridge-needle unit

Holder

Ribbed collar

Plunger rod

ropine and lidocaine, come in this type of prefilled syringe.

To prepare a closed-system device, hold the drug chamber in one hand and the syringe and needle in the other. Flip the protective caps off both ends. Insert the drug chamber into the syringe section. Then remove the needle cap and expel air and extra medication.

Types of needles

Five types of needles are used to inject drugs: intradermal, subcutaneous, intramuscular, intravenous, and filter. (See *Choosing the right needle*.) Each type of needle is designed for a different purpose.

Before you give that drug

Choosing the right needle

When choosing a needle, consider its purpose as well as its gauge, bevel, and length. Use the following selection guide to choose the right needles for your patients.

Intradermal needles
These needles are $\frac{3}{8}$″ to $\frac{5}{8}$″ long, usually have short bevels, and are 25G in diameter.

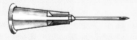

Subcutaneous needles
These needles are $\frac{1}{2}$″ to $\frac{7}{8}$″ long, have medium bevels, and are 23G to 25G in diameter.

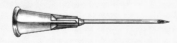

Intramuscular needles
These needles are 1″ to 3″ long, have medium bevels, and are 18G to 23G in diameter.

Intravenous needle
These needles are 1″ to 3″ long, have long bevels, and are 14G to 25G in diameter.

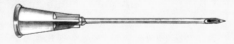

Filter needles
These needles which shouldn't be used for injections, are $1\frac{1}{2}$″ long, have medium bevels, and are 20G in diameter. Microscopic pieces of rubber or glass can enter the solution when you puncture the diaphragm of a vial with a needle or snap open an ampule. You can use a filter needle with a screening device in the hub to remove minute particles of foreign material from a solution.

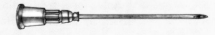

When choosing a needle, consider the gauge, bevel, and length:
• Gauge refers to the inside diameter of the needle; the smaller the gauge, the larger the diameter. For example, a 14G needle has a larger diameter than a 25G needle.
• Bevel refers to the angle at which the needle tip is opened. The bevel may be short, medium, or long.
• Length describes the distance from needle tip to needle hub. It ranges from 3/8″ to 3″.

Real world problems

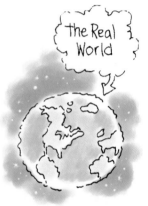

The examples below show how to use the proportion method to calculate doses given by injection.

Prefilled painkiller problem

The doctor prescribes *4 mg of I.M. morphine every 3 hours* for your patient's pain. The drug is available in a prefilled syringe containing 10 mg of morphine/1 ml. How many milliliters of morphine should you waste?
Here's how to solve this problem using fractions:
• Set up the first fraction using the known morphine dose:

$$\frac{10 \text{ mg}}{1 \text{ ml}}$$

• Set up the second fraction with the desired dose and the unknown amount of morphine:

$$\frac{4 \text{ mg}}{X \text{ ml}}$$

• Put these fractions into a proportion:

$$\frac{10 \text{ mg}}{1 \text{ ml}} = \frac{4 \text{ mg}}{X \text{ ml}}$$

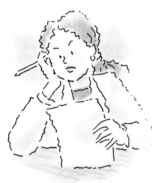

• Cross-multiply the fractions:

$$10 \text{ mg} \times X \text{ ml} = 4 \text{ mg} \times 1 \text{ ml}$$

• Solve for X by dividing each side of the equation by 10 mg and canceling units that appear in both the numerator and denominator:

$$\frac{10\text{ mg} \times X\text{ ml}}{10\text{ mg}} = \frac{4\text{ mg} \times 1\text{ ml}}{10\text{ mg}}$$

$$X = \frac{4\text{ ml}}{10}$$

$$X = 0.4\text{ ml}$$

• The amount of morphine to give the patient is 0.4 ml. To calculate the amount to be wasted, subtract the ordered dose from the entire contents of the syringe:

$$\begin{array}{rl} 1.0\text{ ml} = & 10\text{ mg morphine} \\ -0.4\text{ ml} = & 4\text{ mg morphine} \\ \hline 0.6\text{ ml} = & 6\text{ mg morphine} \end{array}$$

The amount of morphine to be wasted is 0.6 ml.

Medrol milligram mystery

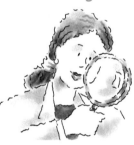

The doctor orders *100 mg of methylprednisolone (Solu-Medrol) I.M. every 4 hours* for your patient with asthma. The vial contains 120 mg/1 ml. How much Solu-Medrol should you give?

Here's how to solve this problem using ratios:
• Set up the first ratio with the known Solu-Medrol dose:

$$120\text{ mg} : 1\text{ ml}$$

• Set up the second ratio with the desired dose and the unknown amount of Solu-Medrol:

$$100\text{ mg} : X\text{ ml}$$

• Put these ratios into a proportion:

$$120\text{ mg} : 1\text{ ml} :: 100\text{ mg} : X\text{ ml}$$

• Set up an equation by multiplying the extremes and the means:

$$120\text{ mg} \times X\text{ ml} = 100\text{ mg} \times 1\text{ ml}$$

• Solve for X by dividing each side of the equation by 120 mg and canceling units that appear in both the numerator and denominator:

$$\frac{120\ \cancel{mg} \times X\ ml}{120\ \cancel{mg}} = \frac{100\ \cancel{mg} \times 1\ ml}{120\ \cancel{mg}}$$

$$X = \frac{100\ ml}{120}$$

$$X = 0.83\ ml$$

You should give the patient 0.83 ml of Solu-Medrol.

Vial trial

The doctor prescribes *100 mg of gentamicin I.M.* for your patient. The vial available contains 40 mg/1 ml. How much gentamicin should you give?

Here's how to solve this problem using ratios:
• Set up the first ratio with the known gentamicin dose:

$$40\ mg : 1\ ml$$

• Set up the second ratio with the desired dose and the unknown amount of gentamicin:

$$100\ mg : X\ ml$$

• Put these ratios into a proportion:

$$40\ mg : 1\ ml :: 100\ mg : X\ ml$$

• Set up an equation by multiplying the means and the extremes:

$$1\ ml \times 100\ mg = 40\ mg \times X\ ml$$

• Solve for X by dividing each side of the equation by 40 mg and canceling units that appear in both the numerator and denominator:

$$\frac{1\ ml \times 100\ \cancel{mg}}{40\ \cancel{mg}} = \frac{40\ \cancel{mg} \times X\ ml}{40\ \cancel{mg}}$$

$$\frac{100\ ml}{40} = X$$

$$X = 2.5\ ml$$

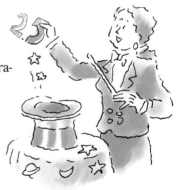

You should give the patient 2.5 ml of gentamicin.

Interpreting drug labels

Before you can safely administer a parenteral drug, you must know how to read its label. Parenteral drugs are packaged in glass ampules, in single- or multiple-dose vials with rubber stoppers, and in prefilled syringes and cartridges.

Looking at labels

Reading the label of a parenteral solution is a lot like reading an oral solution label. (See *A close look at labels*.) Here's the information you'll see:
- trade name
- generic name
- total volume of solution in the container
- dose strength or concentration (drug dose present in a volume of solution)
- expiration date
- special instructions, as needed.

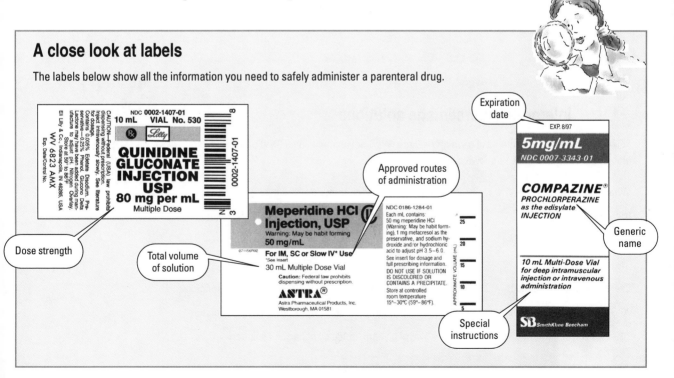

A close look at labels

The labels below show all the information you need to safely administer a parenteral drug.

Percentage and ratio solutions

A solute is a liquid or solid form of a drug. A solution is a liquid that contains a solute dissolved in a diluent or solvent, most often sterile water. Normal saline solution is a solution of salt (the solute) in purified water (the solvent). Solutions come in different strengths, which are expressed on the drug label as percentage solutions or ratio solutions.

Perusing percentages

The clearest and most common way to label or describe a solution is as a percentage. (See *Interpreting percentage solutions*.) Providing information in percentages makes it easy to make dosage calculations, dilutions, or alterations.

On the label, a solution may be expressed as weight per volume or volume per volume.

Weight indicates grams

In a weight per volume solution, the percentage or strength refers to the number of grams — the weight — of solute per 100 ml — the volume — of finished (reconstituted) solution.

> Once again, reading the label is the key.

What does it all mean?

Interpreting percentage solutions

You can determine the contents of a weight/volume (W/V) or volume/volume (V/V) percentage solution by reading the label, as shown below.

What the label says	What the solution contains
0.9% (W/V) NaCl	0.9 g of sodium chloride in 100 ml of finished solution
5% (W/V) boric acid solution	5 g of boric acid in 100 ml of finished solution
5% (W/V) dextrose	5 g of dextrose in 100 ml of finished solution
2% (V/V) hydrogen peroxide	2 ml of hydrogen peroxide in 100 ml of finished solution
70% (V/V) isopropyl alcohol	70 ml of isopropyl alcohol in 100 ml of finished solution
10% (V/V) glycerin	10 ml of glycerin in 100 ml of finished solution

Volume indicates milliliters

In a volume per volume solution, the percentage refers to the number of milliliters of solute per 100 ml of finished solution.

Say it with an equation

Here's how to express these two relationships mathematically:

$$\% = \frac{\text{weight}}{\text{volume}} = \text{grams solute/100 ml finished solution}$$

$$\% = \frac{\text{volume}}{\text{volume}} = \text{milliliters solute/100 ml finished solution}$$

Reviewing ratios

Another way to label or describe a solution is as a ratio. (See *Interpreting ratio solutions.*) The strength of a ratio solution usually is expressed as two numbers separated by a colon. In a weight per volume solution, the first number signifies the amount of a drug in grams. In a volume per volume solution, the first number signifies the amount of drug in milliliters. The second number signifies the volume of finished solution in milliliters.

This relationship is expressed as:

Ratio = amount of drug : amount of finished solution

What does it all mean?

Interpreting ratio solutions

You can determine the contents of a weight : volume (W : V) or volume : volume (V : V) ratio solution from the label, as shown below.

What the label says	What the solution contains
benzalkonium chloride 1 : 750 (W : V)	1 g of benzalkonium chloride in 750 ml of finished solution
silver nitrate 1 : 100 (W : V)	1 g of silver nitrate in 100 ml of finished solution
hydrogen peroxide 2 : 100 (V : V)	2 ml of hydrogen peroxide in 100 ml of finished solution
glycerin 10 : 100 (V : V)	10 ml of glycerin in 100 ml of finished solution

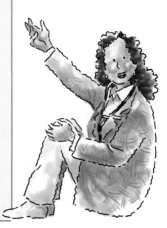

Insulin and insulin therapy

Some drugs, such as insulin, heparin, and penicillin G, are measured in units. The unit system is based on an international standard of drug potency, not on weight. The number of units appears on the drug label. (See *Look for the unit label*.)

Insulin, a potent hormone that's produced by the pancreas, regulates carbohydrate metabolism. The effect of insulin's activity is reflected in blood glucose levels. A lack of insulin causes diabetes.

Insulin injections

Insulin is injected S.C. in patients with chronic diabetes, or I.V. in patients with acute diabetic ketoacidosis. You must calculate and administer insulin doses carefully because a small error can cause a hypoglycemic or hyperglycemic reaction.

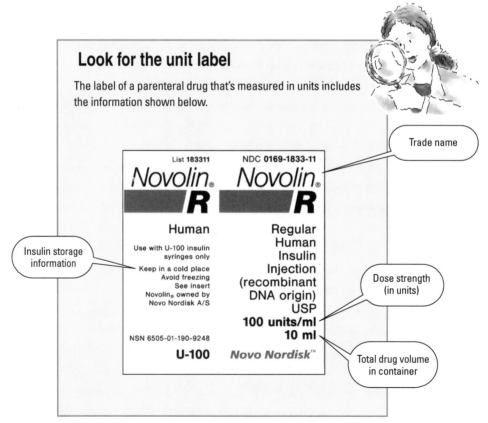

Look for the unit label

The label of a parenteral drug that's measured in units includes the information shown below.

Trade name

Insulin storage information

List **183311**   NDC **0169-1833-11**

Novolin®   *Novolin*®

R   **R**

Human   Regular Human Insulin Injection (recombinant DNA origin) USP

Use with U-100 insulin syringes only

Keep in a cold place
Avoid freezing
See insert
Novolin® owned by
Novo Nordisk A/S

100 units/ml
10 ml

NSN 6505-01-190-9248

U-100   *Novo Nordisk*™

Dose strength (in units)

Total drug volume in container

Types of diabetes

Two major types of diabetes exist: insulin-dependent diabetes mellitus, or type I, and non-insulin-dependent diabetes mellitus, or type II. Type I diabetes typically is diagnosed before age 20 and requires long-term insulin therapy. Type II diabetes usually is diagnosed after age 40 and can be controlled by diet and oral antidiabetic agents, although insulin may be used occasionally to stabilize blood glucose levels.

Types of insulin

Several types of insulin are available. The doctor chooses a particular type based on the patient's diet and activity level and the severity of pancreatic disease.

Insulin origins

Insulin is classified according to its origin (human or animal) and action time. Some insulins are derived from beef or pork pancreas and differ from human insulin by only two amino acids. Others are identical to human insulin and are produced by the enzymatic conversion of pork insulin or by recombinant deoxyribonucleic acid techniques. The origin appears on the drug label.

Insulin initials

The insulin label also contains an initial after the trade name, indicating the type of insulin. These different types of insulin vary with regard to onset, peak, and duration of action. The initials are:
- R for regular insulin
- L for lente insulin
- U for ultralente insulin
- N for neutral protamine Hagedorn (NPH) insulin
- S for semilente insulin
- PZ for protamine zinc insulin. (See *Reading insulin labels*, page 184, and *Identifying insulin subtypes*, page 185.)

Each in its own time

Insulin preparations are modified by combination with larger, insoluble protein molecules to slow absorption and prolong activity. Thus, the different types of insulin vary with regard to pharmacokinetic properties. The following list describes the types of insulin in greater detail:

- *Regular insulin:* also called regular crystalline insulin; insulin precipitated with zinc at a neutral pH; the only insulin that can be administered I.V.
- *Lente insulin:* also called insulin zinc suspension; consists of 70% ultralente insulin and 30% semilente insulin
- *Ultralente insulin:* also called extended insulin zinc suspension; consists of large insulin crystals with a high zinc content in a sodium acetate–sodium chloride solution
- *NPH:* also called isophane insulin suspension; an insulin in crystalline form with protamine and zinc
- *Semilente insulin:* also called prompt insulin zinc suspension; a noncrystalline insulin precipitated at a high pH
- *PZI:* protamine, zinc, and insulin solution. (See *Insulin action times,* page 186.)

What dose do U want?

Insulin doses, expressed in units, are available in three concentrations. U-100 insulin, which contains 100 U of in-

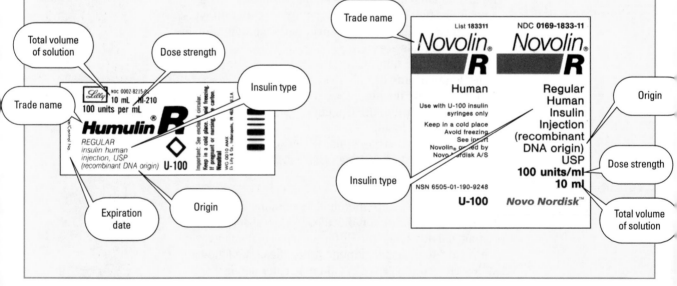

Before you give that drug

Reading insulin labels

Read insulin labels carefully to find the information you need for safe administration. Note that the origin or source of insulin is printed on every label.

sulin per milliliter, is called "universal" because it's the most common concentration. U-40 insulin, which contains 40 U/ml, is a weaker solution that's commonly used by older patients. U-500 insulin, which contains 500 U/ml, is used on rare occasions when a patient needs an unusually large dose.

Before you give that drug

Identifying insulin subtypes

Insulin labels require careful reading because they may contain confusingly similar information. Remember that one type of insulin, such as lente, may come in different subtypes, but that subtypes are not interchangeable. For example, if the doctor prescribes lente human insulin zinc suspension, do not substitute lente insulin zinc suspension USP. Otherwise a hypersensitive patient could develop a severe allergic reaction.

Type	Subtype
Lente	• Lente human insulin zinc suspension (semisynthetic) • Lente insulin, insulin zinc suspension USP (beef) • Lente purified pork insulin zinc suspension USP
NPH	• NPH human insulin isophane suspension USP • NPH insulin, isophane insulin suspension USP (beef) • NPH purified pork isophane insulin suspension USP • 70% NPH, human insulin isophane suspension and 30% regular, human insulin injection (semisynthetic)
Regular	• Regular human insulin injection (semisynthetic) USP • Regular insulin, insulin injection USP (pork) • Regular purified pork insulin injection USP
Semilente	• Semilente insulin, prompt insulin zinc suspension USP (beef) • Semilente purified pork prompt insulin zinc suspension USP
Ultralente	• Ultralente insulin, extended insulin zinc suspension USP (beef) • Ultralente purified beef extended insulin zinc suspension USP

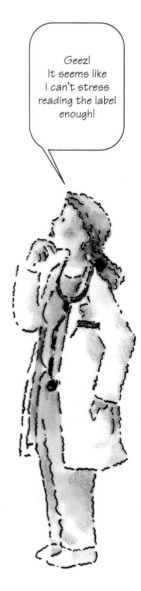

Geez! It seems like I can't stress reading the label enough!

Syringe selection

You need to choose an insulin syringe that's compatible with the strength of insulin to be administered. (See *Selecting an insulin syringe*.) For example, U-100 insulin requires a U-100 syringe, U-40 insulin requires a U-40 syringe, and U-500 insulin requires a U-500 syringe.

A U-100 syringe is calibrated so 1 ml holds 100 U of insulin, a U-40 syringe is calibrated so 1 ml holds 40 U of insulin, and so on. A low-dose U-100 syringe is also used for some patients. This syringe holds 50 U of insulin or less.

Reading insulin orders

Some patients' insulin doses are based on home monitoring of blood glucose values with glucometers. But when a

Insulin action times

Insulin preparations are modified through combination with larger insoluble protein molecules to slow absorption and prolong activity. An insulin preparation may be rapid acting, intermediate acting, or long acting, as shown in the table below.

Drug	Onset	Peak	Duration
Rapid acting			
prompt insulin zinc suspension (semilente)	$\frac{1}{2}$ to $1\frac{1}{2}$ hr	5 to 10 hr	12 to 16 hr
regular insulin	$\frac{1}{2}$ to 1 hr	2 to 4 hr	6 to 8 hr
Intermediate acting			
insulin zinc suspension (lente)	1 to $2\frac{1}{2}$ hr	7 to 15 hr	22 to 26 hr
isophane insulin suspension (NPH)	1 to $1\frac{1}{2}$ hr	8 to 12 hr	18 to 24 hr
Long acting			
extended insulin zinc suspension (ultralente)	4 to 8 hr	10 to 30 hr	> 36 hr
protamine zinc insulin suspension (PZI)	4 to 8 hr	14 to 20 hr	36 hr

diagnosis of diabetes is first made, the patient undergoes tests to determine blood and urine glucose levels. Usually, the patient is enrolled in an outpatient center where he can be educated about diet, exercise, monitoring blood glucose levels and administering insulin. Blood and urine glucose baselines are established.

Based on these determinations, the doctor may order small doses of rapid-acting insulin at set times, such as every 4 hours or before meals and at bedtime, for several days. After a stable 24-hour dosage has been determined, the doctor may order dosage adjustments, such as one or two daily doses of intermediate-acting insulin, possibly accompanied by small doses of rapid-acting insulin.

Insulin on a sliding scale

For a newly diagnosed, ill, or unstable diabetic patient, the doctor may write an order on a sliding scale. This type of order individualizes the insulin doses and administration times according to the patient's age, activity level, work habits, desired degree of blood glucose level control, and response to insulin preparations.

Selecting an insulin syringe

These two syringes are examples of the different dose-specific insulin syringes that are available. The U-100 syringe delivers up to 100 U of insulin. The low-dose syringe delivers 50 U of U-100 insulin.

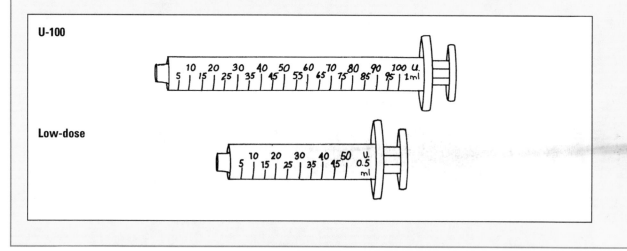

Here's an example of such an order:

Start regular insulin sliding scale:

Blood glucose values:	Insulin dose:
<180 mg/dl	*No insulin*
180 to 240 mg/dl	*10 U regular insulin S.C.*
241 to 400 mg/dl	*20 U regular insulin S.C.*
> 400 mg/dl	*Call doctor for orders.*

Follow the dots

When reading insulin orders, check closely for decimal points that indicate unusual doses. (See *Danger! Disappearing decimal points.*)

If an order doesn't include the dose strength, then administer U-100 insulin, the universal strength. If U-40 or U-500 insulin is needed, the doctor specifies this on the order.

Combining insulins

Regular insulin and NPH insulin are usually given at the same time. When you receive an order for these drugs, draw them up into the same syringe, following this procedure:

1 Read the insulin order carefully.

2 Read the vial labels carefully, noting the type, concentration, source, and expiration date of the drugs.

3 Roll the NPH vial between your palms to mix it thoroughly.

4 Choose the appropriate syringe.

5 Clean the tops of both vials with alcohol swabs.

6 7 Inject air into the NPH vial equal to the amount of insulin you need to give. Withdraw the needle and syringe, but don't withdraw any NPH insulin.

8 9 Inject into the regular insulin vial an amount of air equal to the dose of the regular insulin. Then invert or tilt the vial and withdraw the prescribed amount of regular insulin into the syringe. Draw up the clear, regular insulin first to avoid contamination by the cloudy, longer-acting insulin.

Memory jogger

If you have trouble remembering which insulin to draw up first, think of the phrase "clear before cloudy." (Who doesn't prefer a clear day to a cloudy one?)

This phrase also reminds you how these drugs work: A clear day seems short, but a cloudy day seems to go on forever. Clear, regular insulin is short-acting and cloudy, NPH insulin is long-acting.

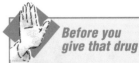

Before you give that drug

Danger! Disappearing decimal points

When reading insulin orders, be alert to the placement of decimal points. Some patients are extremely sensitive to insulin, requiring a dose less than 10 U. To clarify this, the doctor may write the dose with a decimal point.

For example, the doctor may prescribe 3 U of insulin and write it as 3.0 U for clarity. If the decimal point is mistakenly lost during your transcription, the patient could receive 30 U of insulin, a tenfold dosing error. *If a dose seems unusually large or small, double-check it.*

Clean the top of the NPH vial again. Then insert the needle of the syringe containing the regular insulin into the vial and withdraw the prescribed amount of NPH insulin.

Mix the insulins in the syringe by pulling back slightly on the plunger and tilting the syringe back and forth.

Recheck the drug order, and administer the insulin immediately.

Real world problems

Before drawing up and administering insulin, heparin, or other drugs measured in units, check all your calculations for accuracy. The section below shows how to use the proportion method and a sliding scale to calculate insulin and heparin doses. (See *Heparin hazards*.)

Help! How much heparin?

The doctor orders *7,000 U of heparin S.C. q12h*. The heparin you have available contains 10,000 U/1 ml. How many milliliters of heparin should you give?

Here's the calculation using ratios:
• Set up the first ratio with the known heparin dose:

$$10,000 \text{ U} : 1 \text{ ml}$$

• Set up the second ratio with the desired dose and the unknown amount of heparin:

$$7,000 \text{ U} : X \text{ ml}$$

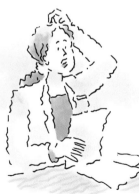

• Put these fractions into a proportion:

$$10,000 \text{ U} : 1 \text{ ml} :: 7,000 \text{ U} : X \text{ ml}$$

• Set up an equation by multiplying the means and the extremes:

$$1 \text{ ml} \times 7,000 \text{ U} = 10,000 \text{ U} \times X \text{ ml}$$

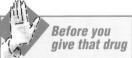
Before you give that drug

Heparin hazards

The anticoagulant heparin is used in small doses to keep I.V. lines patent, in moderate doses to prevent thrombosis and embolism, and in large doses to treat these disorders. Make sure that the heparin concentration is appropriate for the intended use.

Dosage calculation errors with heparin can cause excessive bleeding or undertreatment of a clotting disorder. Remember that the concentration of a heparin flush shouldn't be equal to that of a bolus. The concentration for a heparin flush is generally 1,000 U of heparin in 1 ml of fluid.

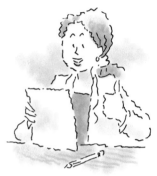

• Solve for X by dividing each side of the equation by 10,000 U and canceling units that appear in both the numerator and denominator:

$$\frac{1 \text{ ml} \times 7,000 \cancel{U}}{10,000 \cancel{U}} = \frac{10,000 \cancel{U} \times X \text{ ml}}{10,000 \cancel{U}}$$

$$X = 0.7 \text{ ml}$$

You should give the patient 0.7 ml of heparin.

Did U say insulin?

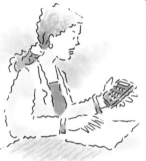

The doctor prescribes *20 U of U-100 regular insulin.* The only syringe on hand is a 1-ml tuberculin syringe. How many milliliters should you administer?

Here's the calculation using fractions:

• Set up the first fraction with the known insulin dose:

$$\frac{20 \text{ U}}{100 \text{ U}}$$

• Set up the second fraction with the unknown amount of insulin and the desired dose:

$$\frac{X \text{ ml}}{1 \text{ ml}}$$

• Put these fractions into a proportion:

$$\frac{20 \text{ U}}{100 \text{ U}} = \frac{X \text{ ml}}{1 \text{ ml}}$$

• Cross-multiply the fractions:

$$100 \text{ U} \times X \text{ ml} = 20 \text{ U} \times 1 \text{ ml}$$

• Solve for X by dividing each side of the equation by 100 U and canceling units that appear in both the numerator and denominator:

$$\frac{100 \cancel{U} \times X \text{ ml}}{100 \cancel{U}} = \frac{20 \cancel{U} \times 1 \text{ ml}}{100 \cancel{U}}$$

$$X = 0.2 \text{ ml}$$

You should give the patient 0.2 ml of regular insulin.

Another dosage calculation under my belt!

Insulin on a sliding scale

Your patient's blood glucose is 384 mg/dl. Based on the following sliding scale (See *How much insulin?*), how much insulin should you give him?

How much insulin?

Insulin doses are based on blood glucose levels, as shown in this table.

Blood glucose level	Insulin dose
< 200 mg/dl	No insulin
201 to 250 mg/dl	2 U regular insulin
251 to 300 mg/dl	4 U regular insulin
301 to 350 mg/dl	6 U regular insulin
351 to 400 mg/dl	8 U regular insulin
> 400 mg/dl	Call doctor for insulin order.

You should administer 8 U of regular insulin.

Reconstituting powders

Some drugs — such as levothyroxine sodium (Synthroid) and penicillins — are manufactured and packaged as powders because they become unstable quickly when they're in solution. When the doctor prescribes such a drug, either you or the pharmacist must reconstitute it before it can be administered.

The strength of one or many

Powders come in single-strength or multiple-strength formulations. A single-strength powder — such as levothyroxine sodium — may be reconstituted to only one dose strength per administration route, as specified by the manufacturer. A multiple-strength powder — such as penicillins — can be reconstituted to various dose strengths by adjusting the amounts of diluent and powder.

When reconstituting a multiple-strength powder, check the drug label or package insert for the dose-strength options, and choose the one that's closest to the ordered dose strength.

How to reconstitute

Follow the general guidelines described below when re-constituting a powder for injection.

Learn from the label

Begin by checking the label of the powder container. The label tells you the quantity of drug in a vial or ampule, the amount and type of diluent to add to the powder, and the strength and expiration date of the resulting solution.

Fluid out exceeds fluid in

When a diluent is added to a powder, the fluid volume increases. That's why the label calls for less diluent than the total volume of the prepared solution. For example, the instructions may say to add 1.7 ml of diluent to a vial of powdered drug to obtain 2 ml of prepared solution.

Say it with an equation

To determine how much solution to give, refer to the drug label for information about the dose strength of the prepared solution. For example, to give 500 mg of a drug when the dose strength of the solution is 1 g (or 1,000 mg)/10 ml, set up a proportion with fractions as follows:

$$\frac{X \text{ ml}}{500 \text{ mg}} = \frac{10 \text{ ml}}{1,000 \text{ mg}}$$

If information about a drug's dose strength isn't on the label, check the package insert. The label or insert will also list the type and amount of diluent needed, the dose strength after reconstitution, and special instructions about administration and storage after reconstitution. (See *Inspect the insert*.)

Check out the chambers

Some drugs that need reconstitution are packaged in vials with two chambers separated by a rubber stopper. (See *Two chambers (One's a powder room!)*.) The upper chamber contains the diluent, and the lower chamber contains the powdered drug.

When you depress the top of the vial, the stopper dislodges, allowing the diluent to flow into the lower chamber where it can mix with the powdered drug. Then you can remove the correct amount of solution with a syringe.

Special considerations

When you reconstitute a powder that comes in multiple strengths, be especially careful in choosing the most appropriate strength for the prescribed dose. (See *One powder, three strengths,* page 194.)

Label logic

Once you have reconstituted a drug, be sure you label it with the following information:
• your initials
• the reconstitution date
• the expiration date
• the dose strength.

Two chambers (One's a powder room!)

Some drugs that require reconstitution are packaged in vials with two chambers separated by a rubber stopper. In the illustration below, note that the upper chamber contains the diluent, and the lower chamber contains the powder. The plunger is depressed to inject the diluent into the powder.

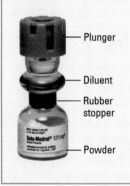

Plunger

Diluent

Rubber stopper

Powder

Before you give that drug

Inspect the insert

The package inserts that are included with drugs often provide a great deal of information that may not be on the outer label. For example, the drug label for ceftazidime provides no information about reconstitution, but the package insert does. Here are the possible diluent combinations as they appear in the package insert that comes with this drug:

Vial size	Diluent to be added	Approximate available	Approximate average concentration
I.M. or I.V. direct (bolus) injection			
1 g	3.0 ml	3.6 ml	280 mg/ml
I.V. infusion			
1 g	10 ml	10.6 ml	95 mg/ml
2 g	10 ml	11.2 ml	180 mg/ml

One powder, three strengths

Many drugs are available in more than one strength. Here's one example:

Nafcillin sodium for injection comes in three dose strengths —10 mg/ml, 20 mg/ml, and 50 mg/ml— as shown below. The availability of multiple strengths allows you to select the one that's most appropriate for your patient's needs.

Less is more

For example, if a patient who must restrict fluid intake needs to receive 1 g of nafcillin sodium, you should choose the 50 mg/ml dose strength because it requires less fluid to reconstitute. As the label states, obtaining this dose strength requires adding 20 ml of diluent during reconstitution. This gives you a concentration of 1 g in 20 ml. You can draw up 20 ml of solution to administer the prescribed dose of 1 g.

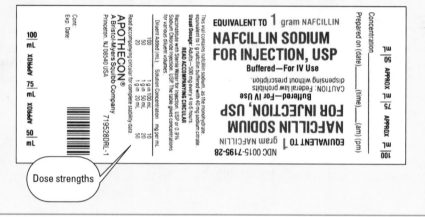

Dose strengths

Real world problems

The following problems show how to calculate the amount of reconstituted drug to give a patient.

Penicillin puzzler (the solution's in the solution)

The doctor prescribes *100,000 U of penicillin* for your patient, but the only available vial holds 1 million U. The drug label says to add 4.5 ml of normal saline solution to yield 1 million U/5 ml. How much solution should you administer after reconstitution?

Here's how to solve this problem using fractions:
• First, dilute the powder according to the instructions on the label. Then set up the first fraction with the known penicillin dose:

$$\frac{1,000,000 \text{ U}}{5 \text{ ml}}$$

• Set up the second fraction with the desired dose and the unknown amount of solution:

$$\frac{100,000 \text{ U}}{X \text{ ml}}$$

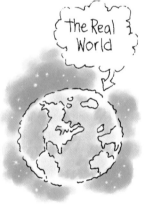

the Real World

• Put these fractions into a proportion:

$$\frac{1,000,000 \text{ U}}{5 \text{ ml}} = \frac{100,000 \text{ U}}{X \text{ ml}}$$

• Cross-multiply the fractions:

$$5 \text{ ml} \times 100,000 \text{ U} = X \text{ ml} \times 1,000,000 \text{ U}$$

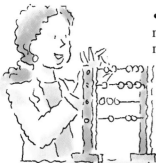

• Solve for X by dividing each side of the equation by 1 million U and canceling units that appear in both the numerator and denominator:

$$\frac{5 \text{ ml} \times 100,000 \,\cancel{\text{U}}}{1,000,000 \,\cancel{\text{U}}} = \frac{X \text{ ml} \times \cancel{1,000,000 \text{ U}}}{\cancel{1,000,000 \text{ U}}}$$

$$X = \frac{500,000 \text{ ml}}{1,000,000}$$

$$X = 0.5 \text{ ml}$$

The amount of solution that yields 100,000 U of penicillin after reconstitution is 0.5 ml.

Deciphering diluents

Your patient needs 25 mg of gentamicin I.M. The label says to add 1.3 ml sterile diluent to yield 50 mg/1.5 ml. How many milliliters of reconstituted solution should you give the patient?

Here's how to solve this using ratios:
• First, dilute the powder according to the instructions on the label. Then set up the first ratio with the known gentamicin dose:

$$50 \text{ mg} : 1.5 \text{ ml}$$

• Set up the second ratio with the desired dose and the unknown amount of solution:

$$25 \text{ mg} : X \text{ ml}$$

• Put these ratios into a proportion:

$$50 \text{ mg} : 1.5 \text{ ml} :: 25 \text{ mg} : X \text{ ml}$$

• Set up an equation by multiplying the means and the extremes:

$$1.5 \text{ ml} \times 25 \text{ mg} = X \text{ ml} \times 50 \text{ mg}$$

• Solve for X. Divide each side of the equation by 50 mg and cancel units that appear in both the numerator and denominator:

$$\frac{1.5 \text{ ml} \times 25 \,\cancel{\text{mg}}}{50 \,\cancel{\text{mg}}} = \frac{X \text{ ml} \times \cancel{50 \text{ mg}}}{\cancel{50 \text{ mg}}}$$

$$X = \frac{37.5 \text{ ml}}{50}$$

$$X = 0.75 \text{ ml}$$

The patient should receive 0.75 ml of the solution.

Attaining the ampicillin answer

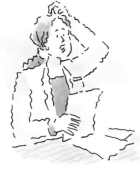

The doctor orders *500 mg of ampicillin* for your patient. A 1-g vial of powdered ampicillin is available. The label says to add 4.5 ml sterile water to yield 1 g/5 ml. How many milliliters of reconstituted ampicillin should you give?

Here's how to solve this problem using fractions:
• First, dilute the powder according to the instructions on the label. Then set up the first fraction with the known ampicillin dose (recall that 1 g equals 1,000 mg):

$$\frac{1,000 \text{ mg}}{5 \text{ ml}}$$

• Set up the second fraction with the desired dose and the unknown amount of solution:

$$\frac{500 \text{ mg}}{X \text{ ml}}$$

• Put these fractions into a proportion, making sure the same units of measure appear in both denominators. In this case, the units must both be grams or milligrams. If you use milligrams, the proportion would be:

$$\frac{1,000 \text{ mg}}{5 \text{ ml}} = \frac{500 \text{ mg}}{X \text{ ml}}$$

• Cross-multiply the fractions:

$$1,000 \text{ mg} \times X \text{ ml} = 500 \text{ mg} \times 5 \text{ ml}$$

• Solve for X by dividing each side of the equation by 1,000 mg and canceling units that appear in both the numerator and denominator:

$$\frac{1{,}000 \text{ mg} \times X \text{ ml}}{1{,}000 \text{ mg}} = \frac{500 \text{ mg} \times 5 \text{ ml}}{1{,}000 \text{ mg}}$$

$$X = \frac{2{,}500 \text{ ml}}{1{,}000}$$

$$X = 2.5 \text{ ml}$$

You should give the patient 2.5 ml of the solution, which will deliver 500 mg of ampicillin.

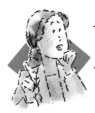

Quick quiz

1. To administer the medication in a prefilled syringe, you need:
    A. a Carpuject or Tubex.
    B. a standard syringe.
    C. dead space.

Answer: A. Prefilled syringes come with a cartridge-needle unit and require a special holder called a Carpuject or Tubex to release the drug from the cartridge.

2. You need to purge a prefilled syringe before administering a drug because:
    A. the cartridge won't work otherwise.
    B. the syringe may contain air.
    C. this ensures needle patency.

Answer: B. You must purge the air from a prefilled syringe. Because a small amount of drug is wasted during purging, most manufacturers add a little extra drug to prefilled syringes.

3. The only insulin that can be given I.V. is:
    A. NPH.
    B. PZI.
    C. regular.

Answer: C. Regular insulin can be given I.V. NPH and PZI insulin must be given S.C.

4. The longest-acting insulin is:
   A. regular.
   B. semilente.
   C. ultralente.

Answer: C. Ultralente insulin has a duration of 36 hours. Regular insulin lasts 6 to 8 hours, and semilente insulin lasts 12 to 16 hours.

5. The needle used for an intradermal injection is:
   A.   26G to 27G and ½″ to ⅝″ long.
   B.   14G to 18G and 1″ to 1½″ long.
   C.   22G and ¾″ long.

Answer: A. A 1-ml syringe, calibrated in 0.01-ml increments, is usually used with this needle for an intradermal injection.

6. In an S.C. injection, the drug is injected into the:
   A.   tissue above the dermis.
   B.   tissue below the dermis.
   C.   tissue in the vastus lateralis.

Answer: B. An S.C. injection puts the drug into the subcutaneous tissue, located below the dermis but above the muscle.

7. A percentage solution can be expressed in terms of:
   A.   weight/volume and volume/volume.
   B.   weight/weight and volume/volume.
   C.   weight/weight and strength/volume.

Answer: A. Percentage solutions are expressed as weight/volume or volume/volume. These are the clearest and most common ways to label or describe solutions.

Scoring

If you answered all seven items correctly, bravo! You've earned the right to say to anyone "this won't hurt a bit."

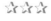 If you answered five or six correctly, congratulations! You're a parenteral powerhouse!

If you answered fewer than five correctly, okay! Remember the golden rule of dosage calculations: Keep things in proportion.

Calculating I.V. infusions

Just the facts

In this chapter, you'll learn:

♦ how to calculate drip rates and flow rates

♦ how to regulate an infusion manually and electronically

♦ how to calculate infusion time and regulate infusions

♦ how to calculate and monitor infusions of blood, total parenteral nutrition, heparin, insulin, and electrolytes.

A look at I.V. infusions

Careful administration of intravenous (I.V.) fluids is critical, especially when dealing with patients who are susceptible to fluid volume changes. Rapid infusion of I.V. fluids or blood products may seriously threaten your patient's health.

To administer I.V. fluids safely, you need information specifying how much fluid to give, the correct length of time for administration, the type of fluid, and what may be added to the fluid. Start by examining the outside of a full I.V. bag and learn to identify all its components. (See *Read the bag*, page 200.)

Next, you will need to be able to select the proper tubing, calculate drip rates and flow rates, and become comfortable working with I.V. equipment such as controllers and pumps. (See *Checking an I.V.*, page 200.)

Getting started

To administer I.V. fluids safely and accurately to your patient, you must select the proper tubing. Selection of I.V. tubing plays an important role in calculating I.V. infusion rates.

Most facilities stock I.V. tubing in two sizes, microdrip or macrodrip. Microdrip tubing, as its name implies, deliv-

Read the bag

The outside of an I.V. bag is an important source of information for calculating infusion rates and times. Read it carefully.

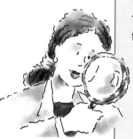

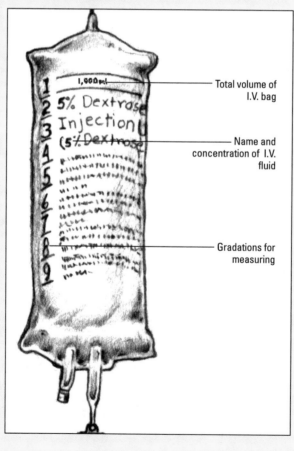

1,000 ml — Total volume of I.V. bag

5% Dextrose Injection (5% Dextrose) — Name and concentration of I.V. fluid

Gradations for measuring

Advice from the experts

Checking an I.V.

You can save time by assessing your patient's I.V. at the beginning of every shift. Performing checks early helps avoid confusion when your shift gets busy.

Are the time, volume, and rate labeled correctly? If so, do they match the order?

Check maintenance fluids and drug infusions, such as insulin, dopamine, and morphine. Are the additives correct? Are they in the right solutions?

After calculating the drug dosage, check the bag again to verify that the solution is labeled with the time, name, and amount of drug added.

If an electronic infusion device is being used, is it set correctly?

Examine the tubing from the bag down to the patient to see if the drug is infusing into the correct I.V. port. This is critical when a patient has multiple lines.

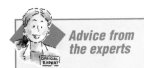

ers smaller drops than macrodrip. Microdrip also delivers more drops per minute. To decide the right size tubing for your patient, you should first understand the purpose of the infusion and the desired infusion rate. (See *Tips for choosing tubing*.)

Targeting the right tube

If the infusion rate for a solution is relatively fast — for example, 125 ml/hour — select macrodrip tubing. If the infusion rate is relatively slow — for example, 40 ml/hour — select microdrip tubing. If you use macrodrip tubing for a slow infusion, maintaining accurate I.V. flow may be difficult if not impossible.

Calculating drip rates

Your next step is to determine the number of drops of solution you want to infuse per minute. In other words, you want to determine a *drip rate*.

To calculate the drip rate, you need to know the calibration for the I.V. tubing you have selected. Different I.V. solution sets deliver fluids at varying amounts per drop. The *drip factor* refers to the number of drops per milliliter of solution calibrated for an administration set.

The drip factor is listed on the package containing the I.V. tubing administration set. For a standard (macrodrip) administration set, the drip factor usually is 10, 15, or 20 gtt/ml (drops per milliliter). For a microdrip (minidrip) set, it's 60 gtt/ml. (See *Quick drip rate guide,* page 203.)

Drip determination

One way to calculate the drip factor is to use the formula below:

$$\frac{\text{Drip rate}}{\text{in drops/minute}} = \frac{\text{Total milliliters}}{\text{Total minutes}} \times \frac{\text{Drip factor}}{\text{in drops/ml}}$$

The three examples below show how to calculate the drip rate using this formula.

Drip rate difficulty

Your patient needs an infusion of D_5W at 125 ml/hour. If the tubing set is calibrated at 15 gtt/ml, what is the drip rate?
• First, convert 1 hour to 60 minutes to fit the formula (we need information in minutes).

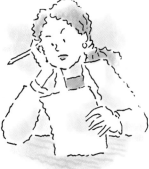

• Then set up a fraction. Place the volume of the infusion in the numerator. Place the number of minutes in which the volume is to be infused as the denominator:

$$\frac{125 \text{ ml}}{60 \text{ minutes}}$$

• To determine X — or the number of drops per minute to be infused — multiply the fraction by the drip factor. Cancel units that appear in both the numerator and denominator:

$$X = \frac{125 \cancel{\text{ml}}}{60 \text{ minutes}} \times \frac{15 \text{ gtt}}{\cancel{\text{ml}}}$$

• Solve for X by dividing the numerator by the denominator:

$$X = \frac{125 \times 15 \text{ gtt}}{60 \text{ minutes}}$$

$$X = \frac{1,875 \text{ gtt}}{60 \text{ minutes}}$$

$$X = 31.25 \text{ gtt/minute}$$

The drip rate is 31.25 gtt/minute, rounded off to 32 gtt/minute.

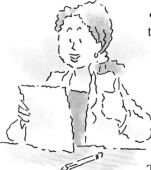

What a drip!

You receive an order that reads *KCl 40 mEq in 100 ml NS over 40 minutes.* You decide to use a controller for the infusion, along with a tubing set calibrated at 60 gtt/ml.
     What is the drip rate?
• Set up the fraction. Place the volume of the infusion in the numerator. Place the number of minutes for the infusion in the denominator:

$$\frac{100 \text{ ml}}{40 \text{ minutes}}$$

• To determine the number of drops per minute to be infused (solve for X), multiply the fraction by the drip factor. Cancel units that appear in both the numerator and denominator:

$$X = \frac{100 \cancel{\text{ml}}}{40 \text{ minutes}} \times \frac{60 \text{ gtt}}{\cancel{\text{ml}}}$$

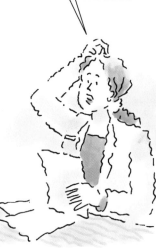

To determine the drip rate, I need to know the drip factor!

• To solve for X, divide the numerator by the denominator:

$$X = \frac{100 \times 60 \text{ gtt}}{40 \text{ minutes}}$$

$$X = \frac{6,000 \text{ gtt}}{40 \text{ minutes}}$$

$$X = 150 \text{ gtt/minute}$$

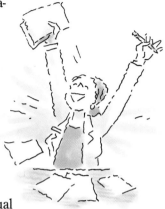

The drip rate is 150 gtt/minute.

Drip rate drill

Your patient needs 15 ml of erythromycin, which is equal to 500 mg. The infusion is to be completed in 30 minutes using a tubing set calibrated to 20 gtt/ml.

What is the drip rate?

• Set up a fraction. Place the volume of the infusion in the numerator. Place the number of minutes in which the vol-

Before you give that drug

Quick drip rate guide

When calculating the drip rate of I.V. solutions, remember that the number of drops required to deliver 1 ml varies with the type of administration set and the manufacturer. To calculate the drip rate, you need to know the drip factor for each product. As a quick reference, consult the table below.

Manufacturer	Drip factor	Drops/minute to infuse (drip rate)					
		500 ml/24 hr	1,000 ml/24 hr	1,000 ml/20 hr	1,000 ml/10 hr	1,000 ml/8 hr	1,000 ml/6 hr
		21 ml/hr	42 ml/hr	50 ml/hr	100 ml/hr	125 ml/hr	166 ml/hr
Abbott	15 gtt/ml	5 gtt	10 gtt	12 gtt	25 gtt	31 gtt	42 gtt
Baxter-Healthcare	10 gtt/ml	3 gtt	7 gtt	8 gtt	17 gtt	21 gtt	28 gtt
Cutter	20 gtt/ml	7 gtt	14 gtt	17 gtt	34 gtt	42 gtt	56 gtt
IVAC	20 gtt/ml	7 gtt	14 gtt	17 gtt	34 gtt	42 gtt	56 gtt
McGaw	15 gtt/ml	5 gtt	10 gtt	12 gtt	25 gtt	31 gtt	42 gtt

ume is to be infused in the denominator:

$$\frac{15 \text{ ml}}{30 \text{ minutes}}$$

• Multiply the fraction by the drip factor to determine the number of drops per minute to be infused (solve for X). Cancel the units of measure that appear in both the numerator and denominator:

$$X = \frac{15 \text{ ml}}{30 \text{ minutes}} \times \frac{20 \text{ gtt}}{\text{ml}}$$

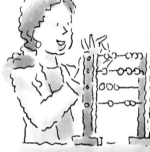

• Solve for X by dividing the numerator by the denominator:

$$X = \frac{15 \times 20 \text{ gtt}}{30 \text{ minutes}}$$

$$X = \frac{300 \text{ gtt}}{30 \text{ minutes}}$$

$$X = 10 \text{ gtt/minute}$$

The drip rate is 10 gtt/minute.

> To determine the flow rate, I need to know the total volume and the amount of time for the infusion.

Calculating the flow rate

If your patient is receiving a large-volume infusion to maintain hydration or to replace fluids or electrolytes, you may need to calculate the *flow rate*. The flow rate is the number of milliliters of fluid to administer over 1 hour. To perform this calculation, you need to know the total volume to be infused in milliliters and the amount of time for the infusion.

Use the formula below:

$$\text{Flow rate} = \frac{\text{total volume ordered}}{\text{number of hours}}$$

For example, if your patient needs 1,000 ml of fluid over 8 hours, find the flow rate by dividing the volume by the number of hours:

$$\text{Flow rate} = \frac{1,000 \text{ ml}}{8 \text{ hours}} = 125 \text{ ml/hour}$$

The flow rate is 125 ml/hour.

Time it for two hours

Here's another example: Your patient needs 250 ml of normal saline solution over 2 hours.

What is the infusion rate?

• First, set up the equation. Then divide 250 ml by 2 hours to find the flow rate in milliliters per hour:

$$\text{Flow rate} = \frac{250 \text{ ml}}{2 \text{ hours}} = 125 \text{ ml/hour}$$

The flow rate is 125 ml/hour.

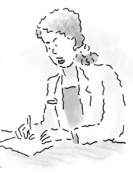

Quick calculation of drip rates

Here's a shortcut for calculating I.V. drip rates. It's based on the fact that all drip factors can be evenly divided into 60.

For macrodrip sets use the following rules to calculate drip rates:

• For sets that deliver 10 gtt/ml, divide the flow rate by 6.
• For sets that deliver 15 gtt/ml, divide the flow rate by 4.
• For sets that deliver 20 gtt/ml, divide the flow rate by 3.

With a microdrip set (drip factor of 60 gtt/ml), simply remember that the drip rate is the same as the flow rate.

Why the microdrip flow rate equals the drip rate

Below is the equation for determining drip rate for a solution with a flow rate of 125 ml/hour (125 ml/60 minutes) when using a microdrip set (drip factor of 60 gtt/ml). Note that the number of minutes and the number of drops per milliliter cancel each other out.

Multiply the flow rate by the drip factor . . .

. . . to find the drip rate.

$$\text{Drip rate} = \frac{125 \text{ ml}}{60 \text{ minutes}} \times \frac{60 \text{ gtt}}{1 \text{ ml}}$$

$$\text{Drip rate} = 125 \text{ gtt/minute}$$

The drip rate (125 gtt/minute) is the same as the number of milliliters of fluid per hour (flow rate).

The shortcut in action

The doctor prescribes *1,000 ml of normal saline to be infused over 12 hours.* If your administration set delivers 15 gtt/ml, what is the drip rate?

• Determine the flow rate *(X)* by dividing the number of milliliters to be delivered by the number of hours:

$$X = \frac{1{,}000 \text{ ml}}{12 \text{ hours}} = 83.3 \text{ ml/hour}$$

• Remember the rule: For sets that deliver 15 gtt/ml, divide the flow rate by 4 to determine the drip rate.
• Set up an equation and solve for *X*. Divide the flow rate by 4:

$$X = \frac{83.3}{4}$$

$$X = 20.8 \text{ gtt/minute}$$

The drip rate is 20.8 gtt/minute or, rounded off, 21 gtt/minute.

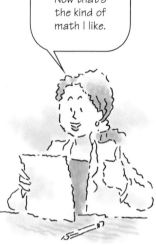

150 ml/hr equals 150 gtt/minute. Now that's the kind of math I like.

Remember the microdrip rule

See if you can solve the following problem without pencil, paper, or calculator:

Your patient is to receive an I.V. infusion of 150 ml/hour using a 60 gtt/ml set. What is the drip rate?

First determine the flow rate. Recall that the flow rate is the number of milliliters of fluid to administer over 1 hour. Simply from reading the problem we see that the flow rate is 150 ml/hr.

Now remember the rule: With a microdrip set, the drip rate is the same as the flow rate. Thus the drip rate is 150 gtt/minute. Just think: You're doing dosage calculations without any math!

Calculating infusion time

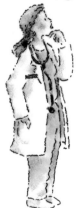

Once you can calculate the flow rate and drip rate, you're ready to compute the time required for infusion of a specified volume of I.V. fluid. This calculation will help you keep the infusion on schedule and start the next infusion on time. It also will help you perform laboratory tests on time, such as the chemistry and electrolyte assessments that commonly accompany infusions.

To calculate the infusion time, you must know the flow rate in milliliters per hour and the volume to be infused. Here's the formula:

$$\text{Infusion time} = \frac{\text{volume to be infused}}{\text{flow rate}}$$

The examples below show how to use this formula to calculate infusion times.

Be back in _____ minutes!

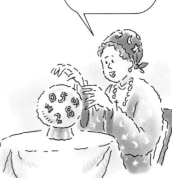

If you plan to infuse 1 L of D_5W at 50 ml/hour, what is the infusion time?
- First, convert 1 L to 1,000 ml to make units of measure that are equivalent.
- Then set up the fraction with the volume of the infusion as the numerator and the flow rate as the denominator:

$$\frac{1,000 \text{ ml}}{50 \text{ ml/hour}}$$

- Next, solve for X by dividing 1,000 by 50 and canceling units that appear in both the numerator and denominator:

$$X = \frac{1,000 \text{ ml}}{50 \text{ ml/hour}}$$

$$X = 20 \text{ hours}$$

The D_5W will infuse in 20 hours.

The bag will be empty at _____ o'clock

Your patient requires 500 ml of normal saline solution at 80 ml/hour. What is the infusion time? If the normal saline solution is hung at 5 a.m., what time will the infusion end?
- Set up a fraction. Place the volume of the infusion as the numerator and the flow rate as the denominator:

$$\frac{500 \text{ ml}}{80 \text{ ml/hour}}$$

- Solve for X by dividing 500 by 80 and canceling units that appear in both the numerator and denominator:

$$\frac{500 \text{ ml}}{80 \text{ ml/hour}}$$

$$= 6.25 \text{ hours}$$

The normal saline solution will infuse in 6.25 hours, which means that the bag will be empty at 11:15 a.m.

An alternative formula

Suppose all you know are the volume to be infused, the

> Good thing I know the formulas for finding infusion time. This thing won't give me the time of day!

drip rate, and the drip factor. Then use the alternative formula below to calculate the infusion time:

$$\text{Infusion time} = \frac{\text{volume to be infused}}{(\text{drip rate/drip factor}) \times 60 \text{ minutes}}$$

Example number one

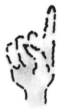

A doctor prescribes *250 ml of normal saline I.V. at 32 gtt/minute*. The drip factor is 15 gtt/ml. What is the infusion time?
• Set up the formula with the known information:

$$\text{Infusion time} = \frac{250 \text{ ml}}{(32 \text{ gtt/minute/15 gtt/ml}) \times 60 \text{ minutes}}$$

• Divide the drip rate by the drip factor. (Remember, to *divide* a complex fraction, multiply the dividend by the reciprocal of the divisor.) Cancel units that appear in both the numerator and denominator:

$$\frac{32 \text{ gtt/minute}}{15 \text{ gtt/ml}} = 2.13 \text{ ml/minute}$$

• Rewrite the equation with the result (2.13 ml/minute) placed in the denominator. Cancel units that appear in both the numerator and denominator:

$$X = \frac{250 \text{ ml}}{(2.13 \text{ ml/minute}) \times 60 \text{ minutes}}$$

• To find the infusion time, solve for *X*:

$$X = \frac{250}{2.13 \times 60} \qquad X = \frac{250}{127.8}$$

• Round off the denominator, and then divide it into the numerator:

$$X = \frac{250}{128}$$

$$X = 1.95 \text{ hours}$$

• The infusion time is 1.95 hours. Convert the decimal

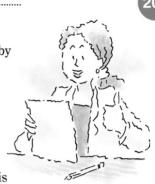

fraction portion of this time to minutes by multiplying by 60:

$$0.95 \text{ hour} \times 60 \text{ minutes} = 57 \text{ minutes}$$

The infusion time is 1 hour and 57 minutes.

Example number two

If 500 ml of hetastarch (Hespan) are infusing at 40 gtt/minute with a set calibration of 20 gtt/ml, what is the infusion time?
• Use the information you know to set up a formula:

$$X = \frac{500 \text{ ml}}{(40 \text{ gtt/minute}/20 \text{ gtt/ml}) \times 60 \text{ minutes}}$$

• Divide the drip rate by the drip factor. Cancel units that appear in both the numerator and denominator:

$$\frac{40 \text{ gtt/minute}}{20 \text{ gtt/ml}} = 2 \text{ ml/minute}$$

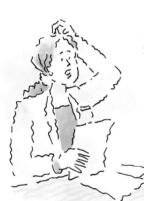

• Rewrite the equation with the new denominator (2 ml/minute). Cancel units that appear in both the numerator and denominator:

$$X = \frac{500 \text{ ml}}{(2 \text{ ml/minute}) \times 60 \text{ minutes}}$$

• To find the infusion time, solve for X:

$$X = \frac{500}{2 \times 60}$$

$$X = \frac{500}{120}$$

• Divide the numerator by the denominator:

$$X = 4.166 = 4.17$$

• The infusion time is 4.166 hours, which rounds off to 4.17 hours. To convert the decimal fraction to minutes, multiply by 60 and then round off the number:

$$0.17 \text{ hour} \times 60 \text{ minutes} = 10.2 \text{ minutes} = 10 \text{ minutes}$$

The infusion time is 4 hours and 10 minutes.

Example number three

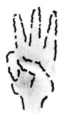

If you infuse 1,050 ml of lactated Ringer's solution at 25 gtt/minute using a set calibration of 10 gtt/ml, what is the infusion time?

• Use the information you know to set up the formula:

$$X = \frac{1,050 \text{ ml}}{(25 \text{ gtt/minute}/10 \text{ gtt/ml}) \times 60 \text{ minutes}}$$

• Divide the drip rate by the drip factor. Cancel units that appear in both the numerator and denominator:

$$\frac{25 \cancel{\text{gtt}}/\text{minute}}{10 \cancel{\text{gtt}}/\text{ml}} = 2.5 \text{ ml/minute}$$

• Rewrite the fraction using the result (2.5 ml/minute) in the denominator. Cancel units that appear in both the numerator and denominator:

$$X = \frac{1,050 \cancel{\text{ml}}}{(2.5 \cancel{\text{ml/minute}}) \times 60 \cancel{\text{minutes}}}$$

• To find the infusion time, solve for *X:*

$$X = \frac{1,050}{2.5 \times 60}$$

$$X = \frac{1,050}{150}$$

• Divide the numerator by the denominator:

$$X = 7 \text{ hours}$$

The infusion time is 7 hours.

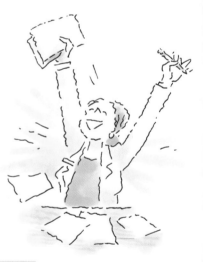

Regulating infusions

Once you start an infusion, you must be careful to regulate the I.V. flow. You can do this three ways: manually, using a pump or controller, or using a patient-controlled analgesia (PCA) pump.

Regulating I.V. flow manually

To manually regulate the I.V. flow, count the number of drops going into the drip chamber. While counting the drops, adjust the flow with the roller clamp until the fluid is infusing at the appropriate number of drops per minute.

One drip...two drip...three drip...four

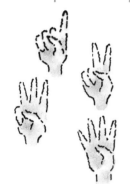

To save time, don't count for a full minute — calculate the drip rate for 15 seconds only. To do this, divide the prescribed drip rate by 4 (because 15 seconds is ¼ of a minute). For example, if the prescribed drip rate is 31 gtt/minute, divide 31 by 4 to get 8. Then adjust the roller clamp until the drip chamber shows 8 drops in 15 seconds.

Afterward, time-tape the I.V. bag to ensure that the solution is given at the prescribed rate and to make recording fluid intake easier. (See *Taped up and ready to drip,* page 212.)

Electronic infusion devices

Electronic infusion controllers and pumps facilitate I.V. administration. (See *Pumped up and in control,* page 213.)

Controllers

Controllers regulate the rate of gravity-fed infusions by electronically counting or measuring drops or by determining the rate based on volume.

Pumps

Pumps administer fluid under positive pressure and are calibrated by drip rate and volume.

A constant flow

When using a controller or pump, set the device to deliver a constant amount of solution per minute or hour, following the manufacturer's directions.

The electronic edge

Electronic devices offer many advantages:
• allowing you to control the infusion rate by setting the volume or drip rate
• shortening the time needed to calibrate an infusion rate

• requiring less maintenance than standard devices that drip fluid by gravity
• providing greater accuracy than standard devices.

Special features

Some pumps and controllers keep track of the amount of fluid that has been infused, helping maintain accurate intake and output records. Many have alarms that signal when the fluid container is empty or when a mechanical problem occurs. Some new devices have variable pressure

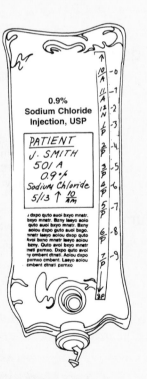

Advice from the experts

Taped up and ready to drip

Time-taping an I.V. bag helps ensure that an I.V. solution is administered at the prescribed rate. It also helps facilitate recording of fluid intake.

To time-tape an I.V. bag, place a strip of adhesive tape from the top to the bottom of the bag, next to the fluid level markings. (This illustration shows a bag time-taped for a rate of 100 ml/hour beginning at 10 a.m.)

0 marks the spot

Next to the "0" marking, record the time that you hung the bag. Then, knowing the hourly rate, mark each hour on the tape next to the corresponding fluid marking. At the bottom of the tape, mark the time at which the solution will be completely infused.

Ink alert

Don't write directly on the bag with a felt tip marker because the ink may seep into the fluid. Some manufacturers provide printed time-tapes for use with their solutions.

0.9%
Sodium Chloride
Injection, USP

PATIENT
J. SMITH
501 A
0.9 %
Sodium Chloride
5/13 ↑ 10 AM

limits that prevent them from pumping fluids into infiltrated sites.

Regulating I.V. flow with pumps or controllers

When using a controller or pump to regulate I.V. flow, program the device based on your calculation of the infusion rate. Remember that these devices can make mistakes — they don't eliminate the need for careful calculations and assessment of infusion rates over time. So check the infusion by counting the drips in the chamber just as you would with manual regulation.

Programming the pump

To determine the pump settings, consider the volume of fluid to be given and the total infusion time. With most devices, you'll need to program both the amount of fluid to be infused and the hourly flow rate. However, some devices require you to program the flow rate per minute or the drip rate.

Pumped up and in control

Infusion controllers and pumps help you control the infusion rate by electronically counting or measuring drops or by determining the rate based on volume. This photograph shows a controller on the left and a pump on the right.

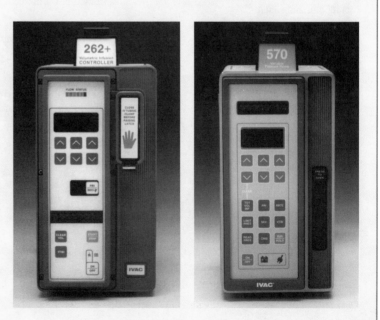

Patient-controlled analgesia pumps

One popular infusion device is the computerized PCA pump, which allows a patient to self-administer an analgesic by pushing a button. (See *Putting your patient in control*.) You program the pump to deliver a precise dose every time. The pump also can be programmed to deliver a basal dose of drug in addition to the patient-controlled dose.

Leveling blood levels

PCA pumps keep blood concentrations of analgesics consistent. With the traditional approach — giving an intramuscular analgesic every few hours — blood levels fluctuate, so patients have periods of heavy sedation alternating with periods of increasing pain.

Two added benefits of PCA pumps are that patients tend to take less medication than they do with the traditional approach and also develop a greater feeling of control over their pain.

Putting your patient in control

A computerized patient-controlled analgesia (PCA) pump, like the one shown to the right, allows your patient to medicate himself with the push of a button. With PCA pumps, patients tend to use less medication than they do with the traditional approach and also develop a greater feeling of control over their pain.

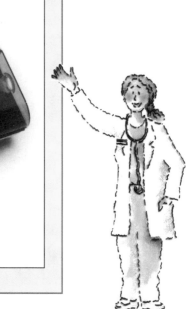

Pump-provided protection

Several safety features are built into PCA pumps. Drug dose and administration frequency are programmed, preventing the patient from medicating himself too often. If the patient tries to overmedicate, the machine simply ignores the request.

Also, some pumps record both the number of requests and the number of times the patient actually receives medication. This lets you evaluate whether the doctor needs to increase or decrease the drug dose.

PCA password

PCA pumps require you to use an access code or key before entering drug dose and frequency information into the system. This prevents unauthorized people from tampering with or accidentally resetting the pump. Some machines even record unauthorized entries.

PCA prep parameters

When preparing a PCA pump for a patient, follow these guidelines:
• Draw up the correct amount and concentration of drug — usually meperidine (Demerol) or morphine — and insert it into the PCA pump. Prefilled cartridges are usually available.
• Program the pump according to the manufacturer's directions.
• Carefully read the PCA log, and then record the information based on your facility's policy. A typical order might state *Start MSO$_4$ PCA. Give 2 mg/hr basal rate and 1 mg/q15 min on demand, with a lock-out of 6 mg/4 hr.*

Regulating drug dosage with a PCA

When interpreting the PCA log, note the strength (number of milligrams per milliliter) of drug solution in the syringe. You'll need this information to calculate the dose received by the patient.

Getting down to basals

Also note the number of times the patient received the drug throughout your assessment (usually over 4 hours). If your patient is receiving a basal dose, note that as well. By multiplying the number of injections by the volume of each injection and adding basal doses, you can determine the amount of solution the patient received.

Multiply this amount by the solution strength to find the total amount of drug, as shown in this equation:

Fluid volume × Solution strength = Total medication received

Record this amount in milligrams in the patient's medication record.

Promoting PCA precision

Most facilities require the nurse who prepares the syringe to record the amount of fluid and drug in the syringe. Each nurse who checks the PCA log double-checks and records this information. The record enables you to double-check the accuracy of everyone's calculations.

Adjusting the infusion rate

No matter how carefully you calculate the drip rate and adjust the flow rate of an I.V., the rate still may change. Why? Perhaps the patient changed position, the I.V. tubing became kinked, or the I.V. became infiltrated. Such factors cause the infusion to run ahead or behind schedule.

Don't hesitate to recalculate the rate

When problems occur, recalculate the drip rate according to the remaining time and volume. If the fluid has infused too slowly, see if the patient can tolerate an increased rate by checking his cardiac and respiratory status. Look for a history of renal insufficiency, pulmonary edema, or any other condition that increases the risk of fluid overload.

If I.V. fluid has infused too quickly, slow or stop the infusion and assess for signs of fluid overload, such as crackles and increased blood pressure. Call the doctor if these occur.

Fluid challenge

You may also need to adjust the infusion rate to perform a *fluid challenge*, protocol for monitoring how a patient tolerates increased fluids. The fastest way to do a fluid challenge is by increasing the I.V. flow rate for a specified time and then reducing it to a maintenance rate. *However, be sure to use a fluid bolus cautiously in pediatric and geriatric patients.*

Heparin and insulin infusions

The doctor may prescribe heparin or insulin to be added to a large-volume I.V. infusion. These drugs may be ordered in milliliters per hour, milligrams per hour, or units per hour. To administer them safely, you must calculate the drug dose so that it falls within therapeutic limits.

Calculating heparin doses

A common anticoagulant, heparin prevents the formation of new clots and slows the development of preexisting clots. Usually given by the I.V. route, it's ordered in doses of units per hour or milliliters per hour. Each dose is individualized based on the patient's coagulation status, which is measured by the activated partial thromboplastin time test.

Flow rate

Accurately calculating the flow rate ensures that the heparin dose falls within safe and therapeutic limits. This type of calculation differs from the flow rate calculations discussed earlier because it's used to administer a drug, not just a fluid.

To calculate the hourly heparin flow rate, first determine the solution's concentration by dividing the units of drug added to the bag by the milliliter of solution. Then write a fraction stating the desired dose of heparin over the unknown flow rate. Then simply cross-multiply to find the unknown flow rate.

Here are some examples using simple proportions to find the solution.

Learning flow rates by example

An order states *heparin 40,000 U in 1 L of D_5W I.V. Infuse at 1,000 U/hr.* What is the flow rate in milliliters per hour?
• First, convert 1 L to 1,000 ml. Then write a fraction to

express the known solution strength (units of drug divided by milliliters of solution):

$$\frac{40,000 \text{ U}}{1,000 \text{ ml}}$$

• Write a second fraction with the desired dose of heparin in the numerator and the unknown flow rate in the denominator:

$$\frac{1,000 \text{ U}}{X \text{ ml}}$$

• Put these ratios into a proportion:

$$\frac{40,000 \text{ U}}{1,000 \text{ ml}} = \frac{1,000 \text{ U}}{X \text{ ml}}$$

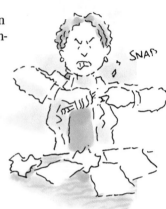

SNAP

• To find the flow rate, solve for X by cross-multiplying:

$$40,000 \text{ U} \times X \text{ ml} = 1,000 \text{ U} \times 1,000 \text{ ml}$$

• Divide each side of the equation by 40,000 U and cancel units that appear in both the numerator and denominator:

$$\frac{40,000 \cancel{\text{U}} \times X \text{ ml}}{40,000 \cancel{\text{U}}} = \frac{1,000 \cancel{\text{U}} \times 1,000 \text{ ml}}{40,000 \cancel{\text{U}}}$$

$$X = \frac{1,000,000 \text{ ml}}{40,000}$$

$$X = 25 \text{ ml/hour}$$

To administer heparin at 1,000 U/hour, you should set the flow rate at 25 ml/hour.

Learning flow rates by example, again

You are about to administer a continuous infusion of 25,000 U of heparin in 250 ml of D_5W. If the patient is to receive 600 U/hour, what is the flow rate?

• Write a ratio to express known solution strength (units of drug to milliliters of solution):

$$25,000 \text{ U} : 250 \text{ ml}$$

• Write a second ratio to describe the desired dose of heparin in relation to the unknown flow rate:

$$600 \text{ U} : X \text{ ml}$$

• Put these ratios into a proportion:

$$25{,}000 \text{ U} : 250 \text{ ml} :: 600 \text{ U} : X \text{ ml}$$

• Solve for X by multiplying the extremes and the means:

$$25{,}000 \text{ U} \times X \text{ ml} = 600 \text{ U} \times 250 \text{ ml}$$

• Divide each side of the equation by 25,000 U and cancel units that appear in both the numerator and denominator:

$$\frac{\cancel{25{,}000 \text{ U}} \times X \text{ ml}}{\cancel{25{,}000 \text{ U}}} = \frac{600 \cancel{\text{U}} \times 250 \text{ ml}}{25{,}000 \cancel{\text{U}}}$$

$$X = \frac{600 \times 250 \text{ ml}}{25{,}000}$$

$$X = \frac{150{,}000 \text{ ml}}{25{,}000}$$

$$X = 6 \text{ ml}$$

To administer 600 U/hour, you should set the flow rate at 6 ml/hour.

Units per hour

If a heparin infusion is ordered in milliliters per hour, you may want to calculate it in units per hour, too. This determines the patient's drug dose so you can be sure it falls within a safe and therapeutic range.
　　Here's an example calculating units per hour.

You use units? Yes, units are useful.

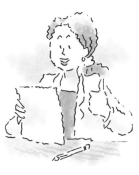

A patient is receiving 20,000 U of heparin in 1,000 ml of D_5W I.V. at 30 ml/hour. What heparin dose is he receiving?
• Write a fraction to describe the known solution strength (units of drug divided by milliliters of solution):

$$\frac{20{,}000 \text{ U}}{1{,}000 \text{ ml}}$$

• Set up the second fraction with the flow rate in the denominator and the unknown dose of heparin in the numerator:

$$\frac{X \text{ U}}{30 \text{ ml}}$$

• Write these fractions into a proportion:

$$\frac{20{,}000\ U}{1{,}000\ ml} = \frac{X\ U}{30\ ml}$$

• Solve for X by cross-multiplying:

$$1{,}000\ ml \times X\ U = 30\ ml \times 20{,}000\ U$$

• Divide each side of the equation by 1,000 ml and cancel units that appear in both the numerator and denominator:

$$\frac{1{,}000\ \cancel{ml} \times X\ U}{1{,}000\ \cancel{ml}} = \frac{30\ \cancel{ml} \times 20{,}000\ U}{1{,}000\ \cancel{ml}}$$

$$X = \frac{30 \times 20{,}000\ U}{1{,}000}$$

$$X = \frac{600{,}000\ U}{1{,}000}$$

$$X = 600\ U$$

With the flow rate set at 30 ml/hour, the patient is receiving 600 U/hour of heparin.

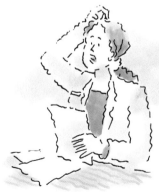

Calculating continuous insulin infusions

An acutely ill diabetic patient may need to receive insulin by continuous infusion. This allows close control of insulin administration based on serial measurements of blood glucose levels.

You'll use an infusion pump to administer I.V. insulin. Regular insulin is the only type that can be administered by the I.V. route because it has a shorter duration of action than other insulins.

Insulin is usually prescribed in units per hour, but it may be ordered in milliliters per hour. In either case, the infusion should be in a concentration of 1 U/ml to avoid calculation errors that may have serious consequences. The examples below are based on common patient situations.

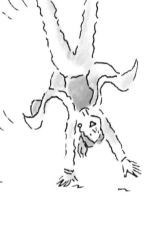

Insulin inquiry #1

Your patient needs a continuous infusion of 150 U of regular insulin in 150 ml of normal saline at 6 U/ml. What is the flow rate?

• Write a fraction to describe the known solution strength (units of drug over milliliters of solution):

$$\frac{150 \text{ U}}{150 \text{ ml}}$$

• Write a second fraction with the infusion rate in the numerator and the unknown flow rate in the denominator:

$$\frac{6 \text{ U}}{X \text{ ml}}$$

• Write the two fractions as a proportion:

$$\frac{150 \text{ U}}{150 \text{ ml}} = \frac{6 \text{ U}}{X \text{ ml}}$$

• Solve for X by cross-multiplying:

$$150 \text{ U} \times X \text{ ml} = 6 \text{ U} \times 150 \text{ ml}$$

• Divide each side of the equation by 150 U and cancel units that appear in both the numerator and denominator:

$$\frac{\cancel{150 \text{ U}} \times X \text{ ml}}{\cancel{150 \text{ U}}} = \frac{6 \cancel{\text{U}} \times 150 \text{ ml}}{150 \cancel{\text{U}}}$$

$$X = \frac{6 \times 150 \text{ ml}}{150}$$

$$X = \frac{900 \text{ ml}}{150}$$

$$X = 6 \text{ ml}$$

To administer 6 U/hour of the prescribed insulin, you set the infusion pump's flow rate at 6 ml/hour.

Insulin inquiry #2

Your patient is receiving a continuous infusion of 50 U of regular insulin in 100 ml of normal saline at 10 ml/hour. How many units per hour is your patient receiving?

• Write a ratio to describe the known solution strength (units of insulin to milliliters of solution):

$$50 \text{ U} : 100 \text{ ml}$$

• Set up a second ratio comparing the unknown amount of insulin to the prescribed infusion rate:

$$X \, \text{U} : 10 \, \text{ml}$$

• Put these ratios into a proportion:

$$50 \, \text{U} : 100 \, \text{ml} :: X \, \text{U} : 10 \, \text{ml}$$

• Solve for X by multiplying the means and the extremes:

$$X \, \text{U} \times 100 \, \text{ml} = 50 \, \text{U} \times 10 \, \text{ml}$$

• Divide each side of the equation by 100 ml and cancel units that appear in both the numerator and denominator:

$$\frac{X \, \text{U} \times 100 \, \cancel{\text{ml}}}{100 \, \cancel{\text{ml}}} = \frac{50 \, \text{U} \times 10 \, \cancel{\text{ml}}}{100 \, \cancel{\text{ml}}}$$

$$X = \frac{50 \, \text{U} \times 10}{100}$$

$$X = \frac{500 \, \text{U}}{100}$$

$$X = 5 \, \text{U}$$

When the insulin infusion runs at 10 ml/hour, the patient receives 5 U/hour.

Electrolyte and nutrient infusions

I.V. fluids can be used to deliver electrolytes and nutrients directly into the patient's bloodstream.

Adding up the additives

Large-volume infusions with additives maintain or restore hydration or electrolyte status or supply additional electrolytes, vitamins, or other nutrients. In such cases, you may have to calculate and prepare the correct amount and add it to the solution.

Common additives include potassium chloride, vitamins B and C, and trace elements. Electrolytes may also be given in small-volume, intermittent infusions piggybacked into existing I.V. lines. (See *Calculating piggyback infusions*.)

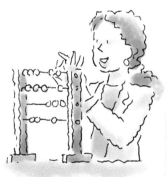

Sometimes, you may need to combine more than one additive into a solution. Before calculating the correct amounts of each substance to inject, check the compatibil-

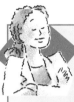

Peak technique

Calculating piggyback infusions

An I.V. piggyback is a small-volume, intermittent infusion that's connected to an existing I.V. line containing maintenance fluid. Most piggybacks contain antibiotics or electrolytes.

To calculate piggyback infusions, use proportions.

Piggyback problem

You receive an order for 500 mg of imipenem in 100 ml of normal saline solution to be infused over 1 hour. The imipenem vial contains 1,000 mg (1 g). The insert says to reconstitute the powder with 5 ml of normal saline solution. How much solution should you draw up? What is the flow rate?

Solution solution

Write the first ratio to describe the known solution strength (amount of drug compared to the known amount of solution):

$$1,000 \text{ mg} : 5 \text{ ml}$$

Write the second ratio, which compares the desired dose of imipenem and the unknown amount of solution:

$$500 \text{ mg} : X$$

Put these ratios into a proportion:

$$1,000 \text{ mg} : 5 \text{ ml} :: 500 \text{ mg} : X$$

Multiply the extremes and the means:

$$1,000 \text{ mg} \times X = 500 \text{ mg} \times 5 \text{ ml}$$

Solve for X by dividing each side of the equation by 1,000 mg and canceling units that appear in both the numerator and denominator:

$$\frac{1{,}000 \text{ mg} \times X}{1{,}000 \text{ mg}} = \frac{500 \text{ mg} \times 5 \text{ ml}}{1{,}000 \text{ mg}}$$

$$X = \frac{500 \times 5 \text{ ml}}{1{,}000}$$

$$X = \frac{2{,}500 \text{ ml}}{1{,}000}$$

$$X = 2.5 \text{ ml}$$

You should draw up 2.5 ml of solution to get 500 mg of imipenem.

Flow rate

Recall that the flow rate is the number of milliliters of fluid to administer over 1 hour.

Compatibility counts

After you've calculated an I.V. piggyback dose, make sure that the drugs to be infused together are compatible. The same goes for drugs mixed in the same syringe or I.V. bag. Drug compatibility charts can be time-savers — you should have one hanging in your unit's medication room. If not, use a drug handbook that includes a compatibility chart.

ity chart or consult the pharmacist to be sure that the additives can be mixed safely.

Prepare to prepare

If the additive isn't prepackaged in the solution, either by the manufacturer or by the pharmacy, you must prepare the correct amount and add it to the solution. Then you must calculate the flow rate and the drip rate. To calculate the amount of additive, use the proportion method as you would for any prepared liquid drug. Here's an example.

Thinking about thiamine

Your patient requires 1,000 ml of D_5W with 150 mg of thiamine/L over 12 hours. The thiamine is available in a prepared syringe of 100 mg/ml. How many milliliters of thiamine must be added to the solution? What is the flow rate?

• Write the first ratio to describe the known solution strength (amount of drug per 1 ml):

$$\frac{100 \text{ mg}}{1 \text{ ml}}$$

• Set up the second ratio. Write the amount of thiamine ordered in the numerator and the unknown amount to be added to the solution in the denominator:

$$\frac{150 \text{ mg}}{X \text{ ml}}$$

• Put these ratios into a proportion:

$$100 \text{ mg} : 1 \text{ ml} :: 150 \text{ mg} : X \text{ ml}$$

• Solve for X by multiplying the extremes and the means:

$$X \text{ ml} \times 100 \text{ mg} = 150 \text{ mg} \times 1 \text{ ml}$$

• Divide each side of the equation by 100 mg and cancel units that appear in both the numerator and denominator:

$$\frac{X \text{ ml} \times \cancel{100 \text{ mg}}}{\cancel{100 \text{ mg}}} = \frac{150 \cancel{\text{ mg}} \times 1 \text{ ml}}{100 \cancel{\text{ mg}}}$$

$$X = \frac{150 \text{ ml}}{100}$$

$$X = 1.5 \text{ ml}$$

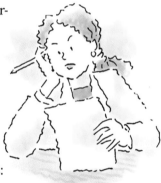

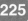
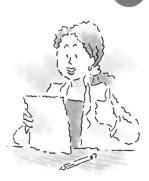

• You must add 1.5 ml of thiamine to the solution. If the flow rate is 1,000 ml over 12 hours, then divide 1,000 by 12 to find the flow rate for 1 hour:

$$\frac{1,000 \text{ ml}}{12 \text{ hr}} = 83.3 \text{ ml/hr}$$

The flow rate is 83 ml/hour.

Blood and blood products

The volume of fluid to be infused and the drip factor can be used for calculating transfusions of blood and blood products. During such transfusions, take care to prevent cell damage and ensure an adequate blood flow by using a special administration set that contains filters to remove agglutinated cells. The drip factor for these sets is usually 10 to 15 gtt/ml.

Generally, you'll use an 18G or larger needle for the I.V. insertion. However, you may need a smaller needle for elderly patients, those with chronic illnesses who are hospitalized frequently, or severely dehydrated patients.

Four hours, max

Your facility probably has specific protocols for infusing blood and blood products. For example, a unit of whole blood (about 500 ml) or packed red blood cells (about 250 ml) should infuse no longer than 4 hours because the blood can deteriorate and become contaminated with bacteria after this time. Many facilities recommend completing a transfusion in about 2 hours. However, this rate may be too fast for pediatric and geriatric patients.

Product precautions

You'll also need to take special precautions when transfusing blood products, such as platelets, cryoprecipitate, and granulocytes. Consult your facility's procedure manual to find out the type of tubing to use and the rate and duration of the transfusion.

In addition, some medical conditions require the use of special tubing. For example, cancer patients may need to use a leukocyte filter with blood products to prevent complications.

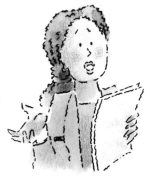

Blood cell brain teaser

Here's an example of a dosage calculation problem that involves packed red blood cells (PRBCs): Your patient is to receive 250 ml PRBC over 4 hours. The drip factor of the tubing is 10 gtt/ml. What is the flow rate in drops per minute?

- First, find the flow rate in milliliters per minute:

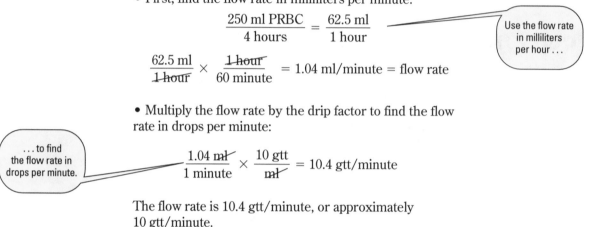

$$\frac{250 \text{ ml PRBC}}{4 \text{ hours}} = \frac{62.5 \text{ ml}}{1 \text{ hour}}$$

Use the flow rate in milliliters per hour . . .

$$\frac{62.5 \text{ ml}}{1 \text{ hour}} \times \frac{1 \text{ hour}}{60 \text{ minute}} = 1.04 \text{ ml/minute} = \text{flow rate}$$

- Multiply the flow rate by the drip factor to find the flow rate in drops per minute:

. . . to find the flow rate in drops per minute.

$$\frac{1.04 \text{ ml}}{1 \text{ minute}} \times \frac{10 \text{ gtt}}{\text{ml}} = 10.4 \text{ gtt/minute}$$

The flow rate is 10.4 gtt/minute, or approximately 10 gtt/minute.

Total parenteral nutrition

A patient receives total parenteral nutrition (TPN) when his nutritional needs can't be met enterally because of elevated requirements or impaired digestion or absorption in the gastrointestinal tract. TPN may also be called central parenteral nutrition or intravenous hyperalimentation.

TPN can be administered centrally through the superior vena cava, inferior vena cava, or right atrium or peripherally through the veins of the arms, legs, or scalp. Most facilities have a written protocol regarding insertion sites and recommended solutions.

TPN is available as commercially prepared products or individually formulated solutions from the pharmacy. Solutions are prepared under sterile conditions to guard against patient infection. Very rarely are nurses responsible for preparing TPN solutions on the unit.

Added attractions

TPN solutions contain a 10% or greater dextrose concentration. Amino acids are added to maintain or restore nitrogen balance, and vitamins, electrolytes, and trace minerals are added to meet individual patient needs.

Lipids also may be added, but they're often given separately to prevent their destruction by the other nutrients. Remember that additives increase a solution's total volume, so they affect intake measurements.

For example, when assessing the amount of fluid remaining in the TPN bottle, don't be surprised to find 20 to 50 ml more than you expected. If this happens, find out whether the volume of additives explains the discrepancy.

The rate goes up...then down

Initially, TPN is infused at a slow rate — usually 40 ml/hour — which is gradually increased to a maintenance level. The rate is gradually decreased before discontinuing TPN. Most solutions are administered through an infusion pump.

For example, a patient's TPN may be increased to a maintenance level of 2,000 ml in 24 hours. To set the maintenance flow rate of the infusion pump, you need to find the hourly flow rate. To do this, simply divide the amount to be infused daily — 2,000 ml — by 24 hours. You find that you should set the infusion pump at 83 ml/hour.

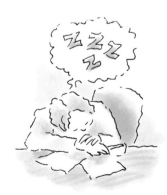

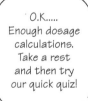

O.K.....
Enough dosage calculations. Take a rest and then try our quick quiz!

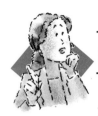

Quick quiz

1. To calculate the drip rate of an I.V. solution, you must first determine the:
    A. drip factor.
    B. flow rate.
    C. size of the tubing.

Answer: A. The drip factor, or number of drops/milliliter of solution, depends on the administration set you're using and is listed on the set's label.

2. An I.V. of 1,000 ml is ordered to infuse over 10 hours at 25 gtt/minute. The set calibration is 15 gtt/ml. After 5 hours, 650 ml have infused instead of 500. To recalculate the flow rate for the remaining solution, you would:
    A. slow the rate to 18 gtt/minute.
    B. increase the rate to 35 gtt/minute.
    C. slow the rate to 10 gtt/minute.

Answer: A. To solve this, divide the time left into the volume left. Then divide the tubing's division factor into the answer and round it off.

3. The test for the therapeutic range for heparin is the:
    A. partial thrombin test.
    B. activated partial thromboplastin time test.
    C. partial thrombin activation test.

Answer: B. Heparin doses are individualized based on the patient's coagulation status, which is measured by this test.

4. For a microdrip set with a drip factor of 60 gtt/ml, the drip rate is:
    A. half the flow rate.
    B. ten times greater than the flow rate.
    C. the same as the flow rate.

Answer: C. The drip rate is the same as the flow rate because the number of minutes in an hour — 60 — is the same as the drip factor.

5. You start a continuous infusion of 150 U of regular insulin in 150 ml of normal saline solution. If the prescribed dose is 8 U/hour, what is the flow rate?

    A. 8 ml/hour

    B. 80 ml/hour

    C. 18 ml/hour

Answer: A. Solve this problem by setting up the first fraction with the known solution strength and the second fraction with the desired dose and the unknown solution strength, putting these fractions into a proportion, cross-multiplying, and then dividing and canceling the units of measure that appear in both the numerator and denominator.

6. The PCA pump can provide a dose of medication on demand or at a:

    A. basil rate.

    B. basal rate.

    C. basic rate.

Answer: B. The basal rate is a continuous infusion administered by the PCA.

7. A fluid challenge is done to:

    A. prepare a patient for an ultrasound test.

    B. hydrate a dehydrated patient.

    C. see how a patient tolerates increased fluids.

Answer: C. The fastest way to do this test is by increasing the I.V. flow rate for a specified time and then decreasing it to a maintenance rate.

8. Putting adhesive tape on an I.V. is done to:

    A. keep the bag from breaking.

    B. make sure the solution is given at the right time.

    C. give you a place to write the patient's name.

Answer: B. Time-taping an I.V. bag also makes recording fluid intake easier.

Scoring

☆☆☆ If you answered all eight items correctly, excellent! Enjoy every gtt of success!

☆☆ If you answered five to seven correctly, great job! Your drip factor is beyond measure! (All right, if you insist, we'll give you 15 gtt/ml.)

☆ If you answered fewer than five correctly, no problem! Go with the flow, keep calculatin', and infuse in peace and joy!

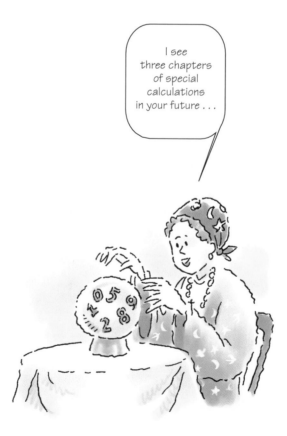

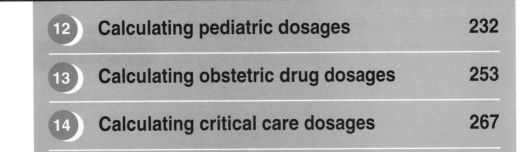

Part VI

Special calculations

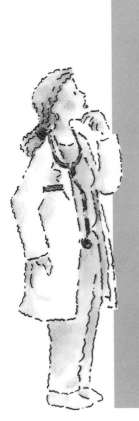

Calculating pediatric dosages

Just the facts

In this chapter, you'll learn:

♦ how to prepare and administer drugs by the four routes

♦ how to calculate pediatric drug dosages according to body weight, body surface area, and Fried's, Clark's, and Young's rules

♦ how to apply pediatric infusion guidelines and protocols

♦ how to calculate pediatric fluid needs based on body weight, calories of metabolism, body surface area, and age.

A look at calculating pediatric dosages

Why is this chapter so important? Simple! Children have special dosage calculation needs.

When calculating drug dosages for pediatric patients, remember that children aren't just small adults. Because of their size, metabolism, and other factors, children have special medication needs and require special care. Also, an incorrect dose is more likely to be lethal to a child than to an adult.

Same routes, different needs

Although both children and adults receive drugs by the oral, subcutaneous (S.C.), intramuscular (I.M.), and intravenous (I.V.) routes, the similarity ends there. The pharmacokinetics, pharmacodynamics, and pharmacotherapeutics of drugs differ greatly between children and adults.

For example, a child's immature body systems may be unable to handle certain drugs. Also, a child's volume of total body water is much greater than an adult's, so drug distribution is altered. Because of these differences, you must be especially careful when calculating special dosages for children. (See *A trio of timesaving tips*.)

Administering pediatric drugs

How you prepare and administer drugs for pediatric patients also differ from the methods used for adults, depending on which route is used. There also are specific administration guidelines and precautions for each route. (See *Giving medications to children,* page 234.)

Oral route

Infants and young children who can't swallow tablets or capsules are given oral drugs in liquid form. When a liquid preparation isn't available, you usually may crush a tablet and mix it with a small amount of liquid.

Remember: Never crush timed-release capsules or tablets or enteric-coated drugs. Crushing destroys the coating that causes drugs to release at the right time and prevent stomach irritation.

Measuring device advice

If a child can drink from a cup, measure and give liquid medications in a cup that's calibrated in metric and household units. If the child is very young or can't drink from a cup, use a medication dropper or hollow-handle spoon. These devices are sold individually and also come prepackaged with some drugs.

Mix it up

If the liquid drug is prepared as a suspension or as an insoluble drug in a liquid base, mix it thoroughly before you measure and administer it. This ensures that none of the drug remains settled out of the solution. Whenever you give an oral drug, check the child's mouth to make sure all of the drug was swallowed.

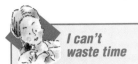

I can't waste time

A trio of timesaving tips

When calculating pediatric dosages, save time and stop errors by following these suggestions:

☝ Carry a calculator to use when solving equations.

✌ Write all the dosage calculation formulas on an index card and keep it in your pocket for quick reference.

🤟 Keep your patient's weight in kilograms at his bedside so you don't have to estimate it or weigh him in a rush.

S.C. route

Pediatric patients also may receive childhood immunizations and drugs such as insulin by the S.C. route. Because the upper arm has the greatest amount of subcutaneous tissue, it's the most common site for these injections. However, any area with sufficient S.C. tissue may be used.

I.M. route

Drugs for pain and sedation and vaccines against diphtheria, pertussis, and tetanus are commonly administered by the I.M. route. When giving I.M. injections, make sure each injection contains no more than 1 ml of solution. Give I.M. injections in the thighs of infants because their gluteal muscles don't develop until they learn to walk. (See *I.M. injections for infants.*)

I.V. route

Fluids and drugs also may be administered by the I.V. route. Because pediatric patients can tolerate only a limited amount of fluid, dilute I.V. drugs carefully and administer I.V. fluids cautiously.

Infiltration and inflammation alert!

Inspect I.V. sites frequently for signs of infiltration or inflammation. Do this before, during, and after the infusion because children's vessels are immature and easily damaged by drugs. If infiltration occurs, stop the infusion and call the doctor.

Keep an extravasation kit handy and make sure you know how to use it. This kit contains drugs and other remedies to treat infiltrations caused by toxic or caustic drugs and helps prevent permanent tissue and vessel damage.

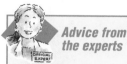

Advice from the experts

Giving medications to children

When giving oral and parenteral medications to children, keep these points in mind:

• Check the child's mouth to be sure he has swallowed the oral drug.
• Carefully mix oral drugs that come in suspension form.
• Give I.M. injections in the vastus lateralis muscle of infants who haven't started walking.
• Don't inject more than 1 ml into I.M. or S.C. sites.
• Rotate injection sites.

Calculating dosages

To calculate pediatric drug dosages, use either the dosage per kilogram of body weight method or the body surface area method. Other methods, such as those based on age, are less accurate but may be used for rough estimates.

Whichever method you use, remember that you're professionally and legally responsible for checking the prescribed dose to make sure that it falls within the safe range.

Dosage per kilogram of body weight

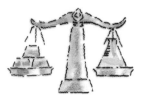

Many pharmaceutical companies provide information about safe drug dosages for pediatric patients in milligrams per kilogram of body weight. This is the most accurate and common way to calculate pediatric dosages. Pediatric dosages are usually expressed as mg/kg/day or mg/lb/day. Based on this information, you can determine the pediatric dose by multiplying the child's weight in kilograms by the required number of milligrams of drug per kilogram.

Shifting weight: From pounds to kilograms

Because most patients' weights are measured in pounds, you must convert from pounds to kilograms before calculating the dosage per kilogram of body weight. Remember that 1 kg equals 2.2 lb.

Peak technique

I.M. injections for infants

When giving intramuscular (I.M.) injections to infants, use the vastus lateralis muscle. Don't inject into the gluteus muscle until it's fully developed, which occurs when the child learns to walk. These illustrations show how to give an I.M. injection using one- and two-person methods.

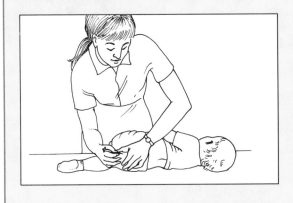

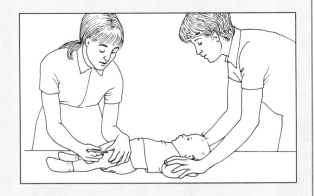

Real world problems

The following examples show how to use proportions to convert pounds to kilograms and how to calculate mg/kg/day.

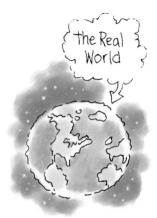

A weighty problem

If your 6-year-old patient weighs 41.5 lb, how much does he weigh in kilograms?

Here's how to solve this problem using ratios:
• Set up the proportion, remembering that 2.2 lb equals 1 kg:

$$X \text{ kg} : 41.5 \text{ lb} :: 1 \text{ kg} : 2.2 \text{ lb}$$

• Multiply the extremes and the means:

$$X \text{ kg} \times 2.2 \text{ lb} = 1 \text{ kg} \times 41.5 \text{ lb}$$

• Solve for X by dividing each side of the equation by 2.2 lb and canceling units that appear in both the numerator and denominator:

$$\frac{X \text{ kg} \times \cancel{2.2 \text{ lb}}}{\cancel{2.2 \text{ lb}}} = \frac{1 \text{ kg} \times 41.5 \cancel{\text{lb}}}{2.2 \cancel{\text{lb}}}$$

$$X = \frac{41.5 \text{ kg}}{2.2}$$

$$X = 18.9 \text{ kg}$$

The child weighs 18.9 kg, rounded off to 19 kg.

Milligram mystery

The doctor orders *a single dose of 20 mg/kg/day of amoxicillin oral suspension* for a toddler who weighs 20 lb (9 kg). What is the dose in milligrams?

Here's how to solve this problem using fractions:
• Set up the proportion with the ordered dosage in one fraction and the unknown dosage and the patient's weight in the other fraction:

$$\frac{20 \text{ mg}}{1 \text{ kg/day}} = \frac{X \text{ mg}}{9 \text{ kg/day}}$$

• Cross-multiply the fractions:

$$X \text{ mg} \times 1 \text{ kg/day} = 20 \text{ mg} \times 9 \text{ kg/day}$$

• Solve for X by dividing each side of the equation by 1 kg/day and canceling units that appear in both the

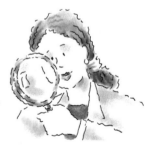

numerator and denominator:

$$\frac{X \text{ mg} \times 1 \cancel{\text{kg/day}}}{1 \cancel{\text{kg/day}}} = \frac{20 \text{ mg} \times 9 \cancel{\text{kg/day}}}{1 \cancel{\text{kg/day}}}$$

$$X = 180 \text{ mg}$$

The patient needs 180 mg of amoxicillin.

A perplexing penicillin problem

The doctor orders *penicillin V potassium oral suspension 56 mg/kg/day in four divided doses* for a patient who weighs 55 lb. The suspension that's available is penicillin V potassium 125 mg/5 ml. What volume should you administer for each dose?

Here's how to solve this problem using ratios and fractions:

• First, convert the child's weight from pounds to kilograms by setting up the following proportion:

$$X \text{ kg} : 55 \text{ lb} :: 1 \text{ kg} : 2.2 \text{ lb}$$

• Multiply the extremes and the means:

$$X \text{ kg} \times 2.2 \text{ lb} = 1 \text{ kg} \times 55 \text{ lb}$$

• Solve for X by dividing each side of the equation by 2.2 lb and canceling units that appear in both the numerator and denominator:

$$\frac{X \text{ kg} \times 2.2 \cancel{\text{lb}}}{2.2 \cancel{\text{lb}}} = \frac{1 \text{ kg} \times 55 \cancel{\text{lb}}}{2.2 \cancel{\text{lb}}}$$

$$X = \frac{55 \text{ kg}}{2.2}$$

$$X = 25 \text{ kg}$$

• The child weighs 25 kg. Next, determine the total daily dosage by setting up a proportion with the patient's weight and the unknown dosage on one side and the ordered dosage on the other side:

$$\frac{25 \text{ kg}}{X \text{ mg}} = \frac{1 \text{ kg}}{56 \text{ mg}}$$

• Cross-multiply the fractions:

$$X \text{ mg} \times 1 \text{ kg} = 56 \text{ mg} \times 25 \text{ kg}$$

First, I need to figure out the child's weight in kilograms, then I can calculate the right dosage.

Next, I determine the total daily dosage.

•Solve for *X* by dividing each side of the equation by 1 kg and canceling units that appear in both the numerator and denominator:

$$\frac{X \text{ mg} \times \cancel{1 \text{ kg}}}{\cancel{1 \text{ kg}}} = \frac{56 \text{ mg} \times 25 \cancel{\text{ kg}}}{1 \cancel{\text{ kg}}}$$

$$X = \frac{56 \times 25 \text{ mg}}{1}$$

$$X = 1{,}400 \text{ mg}$$

Next, I determine the dose to administer every 6 hours.

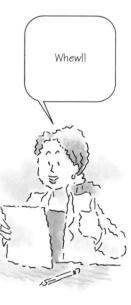

• The child's daily dosage is 1,400 mg. Now, divide the daily dosage by 4 doses to determine the dose to administer every 6 hours:

$$X = \frac{1{,}400 \text{ mg}}{4 \text{ doses}}$$

$$X = 350 \text{ mg/dose}$$

Finally, I determine the volume to give for each dose.

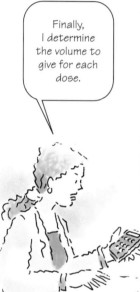

• The child should receive 350 mg every 6 hours. Finally, calculate the volume to give for each dose by setting up a proportion with the unknown volume and the amount in one dose on one side and the available dose on the other side:

$$\frac{X \text{ ml}}{350 \text{ mg}} = \frac{5 \text{ ml}}{125 \text{ mg}}$$

• Cross-multiply the fractions:

$$X \text{ ml} \times 125 \text{ mg} = 5 \text{ ml} \times 350 \text{ mg}$$

Whew!!

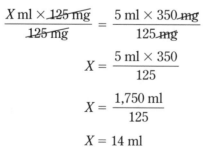

•Solve for *X* by dividing each side of the equation by 125 mg and canceling units that appear in both the numerator and denominator:

$$\frac{X \text{ ml} \times \cancel{125 \text{ mg}}}{\cancel{125 \text{ mg}}} = \frac{5 \text{ ml} \times 350 \cancel{\text{ mg}}}{125 \cancel{\text{ mg}}}$$

$$X = \frac{5 \text{ ml} \times 350}{125}$$

$$X = \frac{1{,}750 \text{ ml}}{125}$$

$$X = 14 \text{ ml}$$

You should administer 14 ml of the drug at each dose.

Dosage by body surface area

The body surface area (BSA) method is used to calculate safe pediatric dosages for all drugs. (It's also used to calculate safe dosages for adult patients receiving extremely potent drugs or drugs requiring great precision, such as antineoplastic or chemotherapeutic agents.)

BSA plot thickens

Calculating dosages by body surface area involves two steps:

☝ Plot the patient's height and weight on a chart called a *nomogram*, to determine the BSA in square meters (m^2). (See *What's in a nomogram?* page 240.)

✌ Multiply the BSA by the prescribed pediatric dose in $mg/m^2/day$.

Here's the formula:

$$\text{child's dose in mg} = \text{child's BSA in } m^2 \times \frac{\text{pediatric dose in mg}}{m^2/day}$$

The BSA method can also be used to calculate a child's dose based on the average adult BSA—1.73 m^2—and an average adult dose.

The formula looks like this:

$$\text{child's dose in mg} = \frac{\text{child's BSA in } m^2}{\text{average adult BSA, 1.73 } m^2} \times \text{average adult dose}$$

Real world problems

The following problems show how these two formulas are used in the BSA method of dosage calculation.

An engrossing ephedrine equation

The doctor orders *100 mg/m^2/day of ephedrine* for a child who is 40″ tall and weighs 64 lb. How much ephedrine should the child receive daily?

• Use the nomogram to determine that the child's BSA is 0.96 m^2.

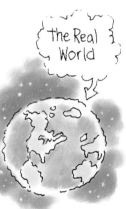

The Real World

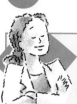

Peak technique

What's in a nomogram?

Body surface area (BSA) is critical when calculating dosages for pediatric patients or for drugs that are extremely potent and need to be given in precise amounts. The nomogram shown here lets you plot the patient's height and weight to determine the BSA. Here's how it works:

• Locate the patient's height in the left column of the nomogram and his weight in the right column.

• Use a ruler to draw a straight line connecting the two points. The point where the line intersects the surface area column indicates the patient's BSA in square meters.

• For an average-sized child, use the simplified nomogram in the box. Just find the child's weight in pounds on the left side of the scale, and then read the corresponding BSA on the right side.

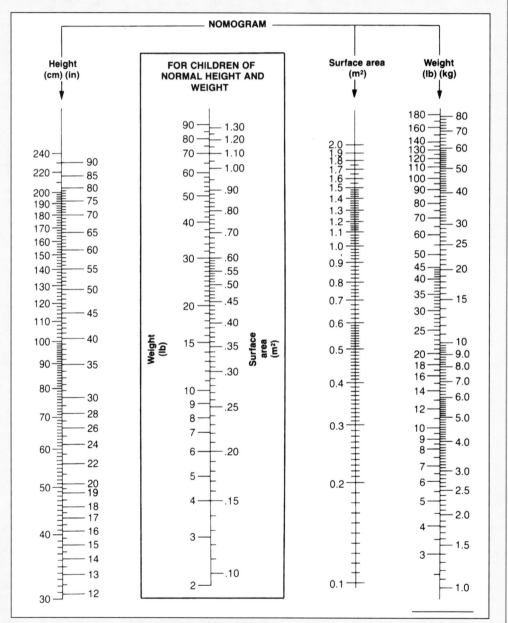

NOMOGRAM

Height (cm) (in)

FOR CHILDREN OF NORMAL HEIGHT AND WEIGHT

Surface area (m²)

Weight (lb) (kg)

- Using the appropriate formula above, determine the daily dosage:

$$X = 0.96 \text{ m}^2 \times \frac{100 \text{ mg}}{1 \text{ m}^2/\text{day}}$$

- Solve for X:

$$X = 0.96 \text{ m}^2 \times \frac{100 \text{ mg}}{1 \text{ m}^2/\text{day}}$$

$$X = 96 \text{ mg/day}$$

The child needs 96 mg of ephedrine per day.

A captivating chemotherapy question

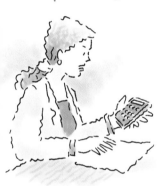

A child who needs chemotherapy is 36″ tall and weighs 40 lb. What is the safe drug dose if the average adult dose is 1,000 mg?

- Use the nomogram to determine that the child's BSA is 0.72 m².
- Then set up an equation using the appropriate formula from above. Divide the child's BSA by 1.73 m² (the average adult BSA), and multiply by the average adult dose, 1,000 mg:

$$X = \frac{0.72 \text{ m}^2}{1.73 \text{ m}^2} \times 1{,}000 \text{ mg}$$

- Solve for X by canceling units that appear in both the numerator and denominator, multiplying the child's BSA by the average adult dose, and dividing the result by the average adult BSA:

$$X = \frac{0.72 \text{ m}^2 \times 1{,}000 \text{ mg}}{1.73 \text{ m}^2}$$

$$X = 416 \text{ mg}$$

The safe dose for this child is 416 mg.

Verifying calculations

After calculating a pediatric dosage using one of the two methods just described, you can further verify the dosages by using one of three other calculations: Fried's rule, Clark's rule, or Young's rule. (See *Verifying dosages*.)

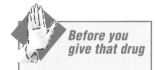

Before you give that drug

Verifying dosages

The three rules below are used to verify pediatric drug dosages. Each uses a different age parameter. It's useful to remember the age parameters so that you know which rule to turn to when verifying dosages for infants and children.

Fried's rule—based on age. Use for infants under age 1.

Clark's rule—based on body weight. Use for children age 1 and over.

Young's rule—based on age. Use for children ages 2 to 12.

Each of these rules assumes an average developmental level for a child, and the pediatric dosage is derived from an average adult dosage. So the results are only approximate. Use them to help verify dosages, not to determine them.

Fried's rule

Fried's rule is usually used to verify dosages for infants under age 1.

Here's the formula (150 months is the age when an adult dose is appropriate):

$$\frac{\text{child's age in months}}{150 \text{ months}} \times \text{average adult dose} = \text{child's dose}$$

Use this formula to solve the following problem.

Fried's rule for infants

The average adult dose of Flagyl is 500 mg. Determine the size of the dose for a 6-month-old child.
• Set up the formula inserting the numbers in the appropriate places and substituting X for the unknown dose:

$$\frac{6 \text{ months}}{150 \text{ months}} \times 500 \text{ mg} = X$$

• Solve for X:

$$X = 0.04 \times 500 \text{ mg}$$

$$X = 20 \text{ mg}$$

The child's dose is 20 mg.

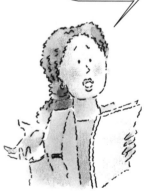

Remember to use these rules to verify dosages, not to determine them.

Clark's rule

Based on body weight, Clark's rule is used to verify dosages in children over age 2. You may use Clark's rule to verify dosages for children ages 1 to 2 because the formula is based on a child's weight, rather than age alone. However, with this rule, the younger the child, the less accurate the dosage.

Here's the formula:

$$\frac{\text{child's weight in pounds}}{150 \text{ lb (average adult weight)}} \times \text{average adult dose} = \text{child's dose}$$

Use this formula to solve the following problem.

Clark's rule for toddlers and tykes

The average adult dose of cefoperazone is 1,000 mg. How much of the drug should you give to your 8-year-old patient who weighs 76 lb?
• Set up the formula inserting the numbers in the appropriate places and substituting X for the unknown dose:

$$\frac{76 \cancel{\text{lb}}}{150 \cancel{\text{lb}}} \times 1,000 \text{ mg} = X$$

• Solve for X:

$$X = \frac{76,000 \text{ mg}}{150}$$

$$X = 506.7 \text{ mg}$$

The child's dose is 506.7 mg, rounded off to 507 mg.

Young's rule

Young's rule is usually used to verify dosages for children ages 2 to 12.

Here's the formula:

$$\frac{\text{child's age in years}}{\text{child's age in years} + 12} \times \text{average adult dose} = \text{child's dose}$$

Use this formula to solve the following problem.

Young's rule for youngsters

The average adult dose of penicillin V potassium is 250 mg. How many milligrams should you give to an 8-year-old child?
• Set up the formula inserting the appropriate numbers and substituting X for the unknown dose:

$$\frac{8 \cancel{\text{years}}}{8 \cancel{\text{years}} + 12} \times 250 \text{ mg} = X$$

• Solve for X:

$$X = \frac{8 \times 250 \text{ mg}}{8 + 12}$$

$$X = \frac{2,000 \text{ mg}}{20}$$

$$X = 100 \text{ mg}$$

The child's dose is 100 mg.

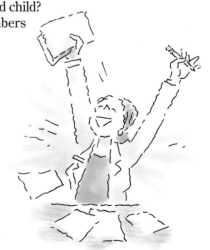

I.V. guidelines

Because pediatric I.V. drug administration is so complex, be sure to follow all written guidelines and protocols about dosages, fluid volumes for dilution, and administration rates.

I.V. drugs are administered by continuous or intermittent infusion.

Continuous infusions

To prepare for a continuous infusion, add the drug to a small-volume bag of I.V. fluid, carefully following the manufacturer's guidelines for mixing the solution. Remember that pediatric patients can tolerate only small amounts of fluid.

Five fundamental steps

Follow these steps to start a continuous infusion:
• Calculate the dosage.
• Draw up the drug in a syringe, then add the drug to the I.V. bag through the drug additive port, using aseptic technique.
• Mix the drug thoroughly.
• Label the I.V. bag with the drug's name, the dosage, the time and date it was mixed, and your initials.
• Hang the solution and administer the drug by infusion pump at the prescribed flow rate.

Intermittent infusions

Drugs given by intermittent infusion usually are infused with a volume-control device such as the Buretrol set. (See *Intermittent I.V. infusion control.*) You also can use a small-volume bag of I.V. fluid with a microdrip set.

Volume control devices have 100- to 150-ml fluid chambers, which are calibrated in 1-ml increments to allow accurate fluid administration. Accuracy is especially important with pediatric patients because children can't tolerate as much fluid as adults and are more prone to fluid overload.

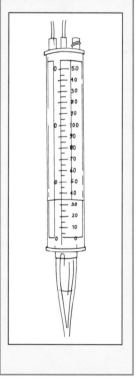

If you're using a volume-control device, follow these steps to start an intermittent infusion:

• Carefully calculate the prescribed volume of drug. Some facilities consider the drug volume as part of the diluent volume. For example, if 100 mg of a drug is contained in 5 ml of fluid, and the total fluid volume should be 50 ml, add 45 ml of diluent because 45 ml of diluent plus 5 ml of fluid drug volume equals a total of 50 ml.

• After careful calculation, draw up the prescribed volume of drug into a syringe.

• Add the drug to the fluid chamber through the drug additive port, using aseptic technique.

• Mix the drug thoroughly.

• Attach the volume-control device to an electronic controller or infusion pump to control the infusion rate. If you're using a small-volume I.V. bag instead of a volume-control device and pump, use a microdrip set, which has a drip factor of 60 gtt/ml.

• Calculate the appropriate flow rate, and infuse the drug.

• Label the volume-control device with the name of the drug.

• When the infusion is complete, flush the line to clear the tubing of the drug. For a peripheral line, use 15 ml of flush solution; for a central line, use 20 ml. Administer the flush at the same rate as the drug. Label the volume-control device to indicate that the flush is infusing.

• When the flush is complete, disconnect the device.

• During the infusion, check the I.V. site frequently for infiltration because children's veins are more prone to this problem.

Calculating pediatric fluid needs

Children's fluid needs are greater than those of adults, so children are more vulnerable to changes in fluid and electrolyte balance. Because their extracellular fluid has a higher percentage of water, children's fluid exchange rates are two to three times greater than adults'. This makes them more susceptible to dehydration.

Four ways to figure fluids

Determining and meeting the fluid needs of children is an important nursing responsibility. You can calculate the number of milliliters of fluid a child needs four different ways:

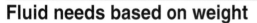 based on weight in kilograms

based on metabolism (calories required)

based on BSA in square meters

based on age.

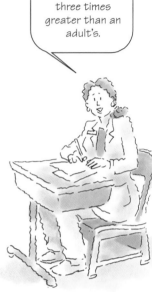

Wow! A child's fluid exchange rate is two to three times greater than an adult's.

Although results may vary slightly, all four methods are appropriate. However, calculating fluid needs based on age is the least accurate method because children vary so much in size at any particular age.

Also keep in mind that fluid replacement can be affected by clinical conditions that cause fluid retention or loss. Children with these conditions should receive fluids based on their individual needs.

Fluid needs based on weight

You may use three different formulas to calculate a child's fluid needs based on his weight.

Fluid formula for tiny tots

A child who weighs less than 10 kg requires 100 ml of fluid per kilogram of body weight. To determine this child's fluid needs, first convert his weight from pounds to kilograms. Then multiply the results by 100 ml/kg/day.

Here's the formula:

$$\text{weight in kg} \times 100 \text{ ml/kg/day} = \text{fluid needs in ml/day}$$

Fluid formula for middleweights

A child weighing 10 to 20 kg requires 1,000 ml of fluid per day for the first 10 kg plus 50 ml for every kilogram over 10. To determine this child's fluid needs, follow these steps:
• Convert his weight from pounds to kilograms.

• Subtract 10 kg from the child's total weight, and multiply the result by 50 ml/kg/day to find the child's additional fluid needs.

Here's the formula:

$$(\text{total kg} - 10 \text{ kg}) \times 50 \text{ ml/kg/day} = \text{additional fluid need in ml/day}$$

• Add the additional daily fluid need to the 1,000 ml/day that are required for the first 10 kg. The total is the child's daily fluid requirement:

$$1,000 \text{ ml/day} + \text{additional fluid need} = \text{fluid needs in ml/day}$$

Fluid formula for bigger kids

A child weighing more than 20 kg requires 1,500 ml of fluid for the first 20 kg plus 20 ml for every kilogram over 20. To determine this child's fluid needs, follow these steps:
• Convert the child's weight from pounds to kilograms.
• Subtract 20 kg from the child's total weight, and multiply the result by 20 ml/kg to find the child's additional fluid needs.

Here's the formula:

$$(\text{total kg} - 20 \text{ kg}) \times 20 \text{ ml/kg/day} = \text{additional fluid need in ml/day}$$

• Because the child needs 1,500 ml of fluid per day for the first 20 kg, add the additional fluid need to 1,500 ml. The total is the child's daily fluid requirement:

$$1,500 \text{ ml/day} + \text{additional fluid need} = \text{fluid needs in ml/day}$$

Use the information above to solve the following problem.

Middleweight fluid problem

How much fluid should you give a 44-lb patient over 24 hours to meet his maintenance needs?
• First, convert 44 lb to kilograms by setting up a proportion with fractions. (Remember that 1 kg equals 2.2 lb.)

$$\frac{44 \text{ lb}}{X \text{ kg}} = \frac{2.2 \text{ lb}}{1 \text{ kg}}$$

• Cross-multiply the fractions. Then, solve for X by dividing both sides of the equation by 2.2 lb and canceling units that appear in both the numerator and denominator:

$$X \text{ kg} \times 2.2 \text{ lb} = 44 \text{ lb} \times 1 \text{ kg}$$

$$\frac{X \text{ kg} \times 2.2 \text{ lb}}{2.2 \text{ lb}} = \frac{44 \text{ lb} \times 1 \text{ kg}}{2.2 \text{ lb}}$$

$$X = \frac{44 \text{ kg}}{2.2}$$

$$X = 20 \text{ kg}$$

• The child weighs 20 kg. Now, subtract 10 kg from the child's weight, and multiply the result by 50 ml/kg/day to find the child's additional fluid needs:

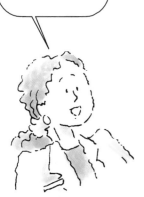

Look closely! I can cancel kg in this equation to find the child's additional fluid need in ml/day.

$$X = (20 \text{ kg} - 10 \text{ kg}) \times 50 \text{ ml/kg/day}$$

$$X = 10 \text{ kg} \times 50 \text{ ml/kg/day}$$

$$X = 500 \text{ ml/day additional fluid need}$$

• Next, add the additional fluid need to the 1,000 ml/day that are required for the first 10 kg (because the child weighs between 10 and 20 kg).

$$X = 1,000 \text{ ml/day} + 500 \text{ ml/day}$$

$$X = 1,500 \text{ ml/day}$$

The child should receive 1,500 ml of fluid in 24 hours to meet his fluid maintenance needs.

Fluid needs based on calories

You can calculate fluid needs based on calories because water is necessary for metabolism. A child should receive 120 ml of fluid for every 100 kilocalories (kcal [also commonly called calories]) of metabolism.

Fluids help burn calories

To calculate fluid requirements based on calorie requirements, follow these steps:
• Find the child's calorie requirements. You can take this from a table of recommended dietary allowances for children, or you can have a dietitian calculate it.
• Divide the calorie requirements by 100 kcal because fluid requirements are determined for every 100 calories.

- Multiply the results by 120 ml—the amount of fluid required for every 100 kcal.

Here's the formula:

$$\text{fluid requirements in ml/day} = \frac{\text{calorie requirements}}{100 \text{ kcal}} \times 120 \text{ ml}$$

Use the information above to solve the following problem.

Calorie-conscious problem

Your pediatric patient uses 900 calories/day. What are his daily fluid requirements?
- Set up the formula inserting the appropriate numbers and substituting X for the unknown amount of fluid:

$$\frac{900 \text{ kcal}}{100 \text{ kcal}} \times 120 \text{ ml} = X$$

$$X = 9 \times 120 \text{ ml}$$

$$X = 1{,}080 \text{ ml}$$

The patient needs 1,080 ml of fluid per day.

Fluid needs based on BSA

Another method for determining pediatric maintenance fluid requirements is based on the child's BSA. To calculate the daily fluid needs of a child who isn't dehydrated, multiply the BSA by 1,500, as shown in this formula:

$$\text{fluid maintenance needs in ml/day} = \text{BSA in m}^2 \times 1{,}500 \text{ ml/day/m}^2$$

Use this formula to solve the following problem.

Cancel m² to find the answer in ml/day.

BSA-based problem

Your patient is 36″ tall and weighs 40 lb. If his BSA is 0.72 m², how much fluid does he need each day?
- Set up the equation, inserting the appropriate numbers and substituting X for the unknown amount of fluid. Then solve for X:

$$X = 0.72 \text{ m}^2 \times 1{,}500 \text{ ml/day/m}^2$$
$$X = 1{,}080 \text{ ml/day}$$

The child needs 1,080 ml of fluid per day.

Fluid needs based on age

A child under age 1 requires 125 to 150 ml of fluid per kg/day. To determine the lower boundary of the range of fluid needed, multiply the child's weight by 125 ml/kg/day, as shown in this formula:

weight in kg × 125 ml/kg/day = lower boundary in ml/day

To determine the upper boundary of the range, multiply the child's weight by 150 ml/kg/day, as shown in this formula:

weight in kg × 150 ml/kg/day = upper boundary in ml/day

Age matters in this fluid formula

A child age 1 or older requires 1,000 ml of fluid per day plus 100 ml/day for each year over age 1 (not to exceed 2,500 ml/day). To determine the fluid needs of this child, follow these steps:
• Assign 1,000 ml of fluid per day for the first year of the child's age.
• Subtract 1 year from the child's age, and multiply the result by 100 ml per day.
    Here's the formula:

(age − 1 year) × 100 ml/day = additional fluid need in ml/day

• Add the result to 1,000 ml/day. The total is the child's daily fluid requirement.
    Here's the formula:

fluid needs in ml/day = 1,000 ml/day + additional fluid need

Use this formula to solve the following problem.

An age-specific problem

Your 2-month-old patient weighs 5 kg. What is the appropriate range of fluid volume that she should receive?
• To determine the lower boundary of the range of fluid needed, set up the following equation and solve for X:

$$X = 5 \, \text{kg} \times 125 \, \text{ml/kg/day}$$

$$X = 625 \, \text{ml}$$

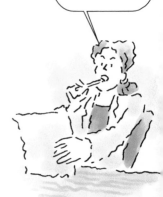

To find this child's range of fluid needs in ml/day, I canceled kg in these equations.

• To determine the upper boundary for the range of fluid, set up the same equation, using 150 ml for the upper boundary:

$$X = 5 \text{ kg} \times 150 \text{ ml/kg/day}$$

$$X = 750 \text{ ml}$$

The patient should receive 625 to 750 ml of fluid per day.

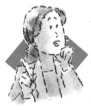

Quick quiz

1. The equation used to convert pounds to kilograms is:
   A. kilograms divided by 2.2
   B. pounds divided by 2.2
   C. milligrams divided by 2.2

Answer: B. To convert pounds to kilograms, divide the weight in pounds by 2.2 because 1 kg equals 2.2 lb.

2. Fried's rule for verifying pediatric dosages is based on:
   A. age.
   B. weight.
   C. BSA.

Answer: A. Fried's rule is based on age only and is used for children under age 1.

3. If the suggested pediatric dosage for a drug is 35 mg/kg/day, the amount to give an infant weighing 5 kg is:
   A. 250 mg
   B. 175 mg
   C. 75 mg

Answer: B. To solve this problem, set up a proportion with the suggested dosage in one ratio and the unknown quantity in the other ratio. Solve for X by multiplying the means and the extremes and then dividing each side of the equation by the value that appears on the same side of the equation as X. Cancel units that appear in both the numerator and denominator.

4. A child who uses 1,000 calories per day has daily fluid requirements of:
   A. 1,000 ml
   B. 200 ml
   C. 1,200 ml

Answer: C. Use the equation for calculating fluid needs based on kilocalories, inserting the appropriate numbers. Then solve for X.

5. If a patient is 40″ tall, weighs 64 lb , and has a BSA of 0.96 m², how much fluid does he require per day?
   A. 1,400 ml
   B. 140 ml
   C. 1,440 ml

Answer: C. Use the equation for calculating fluid needs based on BSA, inserting the appropriate numbers. Then solve for X.

6. If the average adult dose of a drug is 250 mg, how many milligrams should you give to a 6-year-old?
   A. 38 mg
   B. 83 mg
   C. 183 mg

Answer: B. To calculate drug dosage based on weight, use the BSA method. Insert the appropriate numbers in the formula, and solve for X. Verify the dosage by using Young's rule which is based on a child's age.

7. The chart used to determine BSA is the:
   A. monogram.
   B. nomogram.
   C. pediagram.

Answer: B. A nomogram lets you plot the patient's height and weight to determine the BSA.

Scoring

☆☆☆   If you answered all seven items correctly, way to go! You're ruler of the rules—Fried, Clark, and Young would be proud.

☆☆   If you answered four to six correctly, we're impressed! You're the pride of precise pediatric dosages!

☆   If you answered fewer than four correctly, review the chapter and try again. You'll be a specialist in special calculations before you know it!

Calculating obstetric drug dosages

Just the facts

In this chapter, you'll learn:

♦ how to assess the mother and fetus during medication administration

♦ the common obstetric drugs and their adverse effects

♦ how to calculate obstetric dosages.

A look at obstetric drug administration

During labor and delivery, drugs are commonly given to the mother for four reasons:

to reverse the effects of pregnancy-induced hypertension

to inhibit preterm labor

to induce labor

to prevent postpartal hemorrhage.

Because drugs administered to the mother also can affect the fetus, both the mother and fetus need meticulous monitoring. *Remember: You're caring for two patients at once, so there's a narrow margin for error.*

Assessing the mother and fetus

When administering medications, check the mother's vital signs, urine output, uterine contractions, and deep tendon reflexes frequently. (See *Assessing the mother's body systems,* page 254.) Assess fluid intake and output and breath sounds carefully to reduce the mother's risk for fluid overload, which can lead to acute pulmonary edema.

Fluid monitoring is especially critical in women with pregnancy-induced hypertension, which can cause decreased renal function. It's also important when drugs are given to inhibit preterm labor because these drugs have an antidiuretic effect.

Don't forget the fetus

While you're evaluating the mother, be sure to evaluate the fetus's response to drug therapy. Constantly assess the fetal heart tones and heart rate by connecting the mother to an electronic fetal monitor. This monitor records the heart rate and also provides a tracing of it.

Be alert for a sudden increase or decrease in the fetal heart rate, which may signal an adverse reaction to treatment. If either of these occur, discontinue the drug immediately. (See *It's got a good beat: Contractions and fetal heart rate.*)

Remember to assess the fetus's response to drug therapy.

Commonly used drugs

Drugs used during labor and delivery include ritodrine hydrochloride (Yutopar), terbutaline sulfate (Brethine), magnesium sulfate, and oxytocin (Pitocin).

Peak technique

Assessing the mother's body systems

Assessment is a critical part of obstetric nursing. Here's what to assess in each of the mother's body systems.

Neurologic system
- Deep tendon reflexes when magnesium sulfate is infusing
- Pain
- Orientation—disorientation can indicate hypoxemia

Cardiovascular system
- Vital signs
- Extremities for peripheral edema with large-volume infusions
- Pulses and skin temperature in the lower extremities for evidence of deep vein thrombosis; also assess for Homans' sign by dorsiflexing the foot while supporting the leg—deep calf pain indicates thrombophlebitis
- I.V. site to prevent infiltration

Respiratory system
- Breath sounds
- Need for oxygen
- Lungs for pulmonary edema with large-volume infusions

Gastrointestinal system
- Abdomen for contractions when oxytocin is infusing
- Abdomen for bowel sounds after delivery
- Ability to move bowels before discharge

Genitourinary system
- Urine output
- Fluid balance to check for decreased renal function

Preventing preterm labor

Ritodrine and terbutaline are used to inhibit preterm labor. These drugs stimulate the beta$_2$-adrenergic receptors in the uterine smooth muscle and inhibit contractility.

To administer one of these drugs, mix it in a compatible I.V. solution and administer it through an infusion pump. Then titrate the dose every 10 minutes until the contractions subside, the maximum dose is reached, or the patient is unable to tolerate the drug due to its adverse effects.

Controlling convulsions

Another drug used during labor and delivery is magnesium sulfate, which prevents or controls seizures that may be caused by pregnancy-induced hypertension. The drug may decrease acetylcholine levels, but its exact anticonvulsant mechanism is unknown.

To administer magnesium sulfate, first give a loading dose, which is a high dose given over a short time. This is necessary to reach a therapeutic drug level. This is followed by an infusion at a lower dose, as prescribed.

During the infusion, closely assess knee jerk and patellar reflexes; loss of these signals drug toxicity. If toxi-

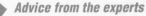

Advice from the experts

It's got a good beat: Contractions and fetal heart rate

While you're monitoring the mother's contractions, assess the fetal heart rate, too. Follow this checklist:

1. Evaluate the mother's contraction pattern.

2. Note the characteristics of the contractions:
- what is the frequency?
- what is the duration?
- what is the intensity?

3. Evaluate the fetal heart rate:
- establish a baseline.
- is rate within normal range?
- is tachycardia present?
- is bradycardia present?

4. Determine the fetal heart rate variability:
- what is the short-term variability?
- what is the long-term variability?

5. Assess for changes in fetal heart rate characteristics:
- is acceleration or increased heart rate present with contractions?
- is deceleration or decreased heart rate present with contractions?
- is heart rate waveform regular and uniform in shape?
- is heart rate waveform irregular in shape?

city occurs, the doctor will probably order calcium gluconate (Kalcinate) as an antidote.

Compelling contractions

Oxytocin — the most commonly used drug to induce labor — selectively stimulates uterine smooth muscle. After mixing it with a compatible solution, administer it by I.V. infusion pump and titrate it until a normal contraction pattern occurs.

When labor is firmly established, decrease the infusion rate. Carefully monitor contraction strength because the drug can cause severe contractions that can lead to uterine rupture and fetal and maternal death.

Blocking bleeding

Oxytocin also may be used to control bleeding after delivery of the placenta. To accomplish this, add the drug to 1 L of I.V. fluid, and then infuse it at a rate that controls bleeding but doesn't exceed 20 milliunits (mU) per minute. (See *The lowdown on four obstetric drugs,* pages 257 to 259.)

Dosage calculations

In the labor and delivery unit, you must be especially careful to calculate and administer drugs accurately. For one thing, you may be dealing with life-threatening problems, such as hemorrhage or seizures caused by pregnancy-induced hypertension.

For another thing, you're caring for two patients at once — the mother and the fetus. Administering accurate dosages to the mother helps avoid fetal complications. Make sure you examine drug labels closely. They contain valuable information for calculating dosages. (See *Learn from labels,* page 260.)

Real world problems

The examples below show how to calculate obstetric drugs using proportions.

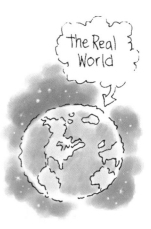
The Real World

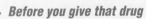

Before you give that drug

The lowdown on four obstetric drugs

This table lists some common drugs used in the obstetric setting along with their actions, adverse reactions, and nursing considerations.

Drug	Action	Adverse reactions	Nursing considerations
oxytocin (Pitocin)	Causes potent and selective stimulation of uterine and mammary gland smooth muscle	**Maternal** • *Blood:* afibrinogenemia; (may be related to increased postpartum bleeding); thrombocytopenia • *CNS:* subarachnoid hemorrhage resulting from hypertension; seizures or coma resulting from water intoxication • *CV:* hypotension, increased heart rate, systemic venous return, increased cardiac output, arrhythmias • *Other:* hypersensitivity, tetanic contractions, abruptio placentae, impaired uterine blood flow, increased uterine motility **Fetal** • *Blood:* hyperbilirubinemia, hypercapnia • *CV:* bradycardia, tachycardia, premature ventricular contractions • *Other:* hypoxia, asphyxia, and death • *CNS:* brain damage, seizures • *CV:* variable deceleration of heart rate • *EENT:* retinal hemorrhage • *GI:* hepatic necrosis	• Contraindicated in cephalopelvic disproportion; where delivery requires conversion, as in transverse lie; in fetal distress; when delivery isn't imminent; and in other obstetric emergencies. • Administer by piggyback infusion so drug can be discontinued without interrupting I.V. line. *Don't give by I.V. bolus injection.* • Don't infuse in more than one site. • Every 15 minutes monitor and record uterine contractions, heart rate, blood pressure, intrauterine pressure, fetal heart rate, and character of blood loss. • Have magnesium sulfate (20% solution) available for relaxation of myometrium.

(continued)

The lowdown on four obstetric drugs (continued)

Drug	Action	Adverse reactions	Nursing considerations
terbutaline sulfate (Brethine)	Relaxes uterine muscle by acting on beta$_2$-adrenergic receptors; inhibits uterine contractions	**Maternal** • *Blood:* increased liver enzymes • *CNS:* seizures, nervousness, tremor, headache, drowsiness, flushing, sweating • *CV:* increased heart rate, changes in blood pressure, palpitations, chest discomfort • *EENT:* tinnitus • *GI:* nausea, vomiting, altered taste • *Resp:* dyspnea, wheezing	• Use cautiously with diabetes, hypertension, hyperthyroidism, severe cardiac disease, and arrhythmias. • Protect from light. *Don't use if discolored.* • Explain need for drug to patient and family. • Give subcutaneous injection in lateral deltoid area. • Warn patient about possibility of paradoxical bronchospasm. • Tell patient she may use tablets and aerosol concomitantly. • Teach patient how to administer metered dose. • Although not approved by FDA for treatment of preterm labor, drug is considered very effective and is used in many hospitals. • Monitor neonate for hypoglycemia.
magnesium sulfate	May decrease acetylcholine released by nerve impulse, but anticonvulsant mechanisms unknown	**Maternal** • *CNS:* sweating, drowsiness, depressed reflexes, flaccid paralysis, hypothermia, flushing • *CV:* hypotension, circulatory collapse, depressed cardiac function, heart block • *Other:* fatal respiratory paralysis, hypocalcemia with tetany	• Use drug cautiously in impaired renal function, myocardial damage, and heart block and during labor. • Drug can decrease frequency and force of uterine contractions. • Keep calcium gluconate available to reverse magnesium intoxication. • Use drug cautiously in patients undergoing digitalization because arrhythmia may occur. • Watch for respiratory depression. • Monitor intake and output. • Monitor deep tendon reflexes. • Monitor neonate for magnesium toxicity. • Maximum infusion is 150 mg/minute. • Signs of hypermagnesemia begin to appear at blood levels of 4 mEq/L. • Drug may be used as a tocolytic agent to inhibit premature labor. • Monitor neonate for magnesium toxicity. • Drug should be stopped at least 2 hours before delivery to avoid fetal respiratory depression.

The lowdown on four obstetric drugs *(continued)*

Drug	Action	Adverse reactions	Nursing considerations
ritodrine hydrochloride (Yutopar)	A beta-receptor agonist that stimulates the beta$_2$-adrenergic receptors in uterine smooth muscle, inhibiting contractility	**Maternal** • *CNS:* nervousness, anxiety, headache • *CV:* dose-related alterations in blood pressure, palpitations, pulmonary edema, tachycardia, ECG changes • *GI:* nausea • *Metabolic:* hyperglycemia, hypokalemia • *Other:* erythema **Fetal** • *Blood:* hypoglycemia • *CV:* increased heart rate, hypotension	• Drug is contraindicated before 20 weeks of pregnancy. • Drug is contraindicated in antepartum hemorrhage, eclampsia, intrauterine fetal death, chorioamnionitis, maternal cardiac disease, pulmonary hypertension, maternal hyperthyroidism, and uncontrolled maternal diabetes mellitus. • Monitor maternal pulse and blood pressure and fetal heart rate. A maternal heart rate over 140 beats per minute or a persistent respiratory rate of over 20 breaths per minute may signal impending pulmonary edema. • Discontinue if pulmonary edema occurs. • Monitor fluid administration to prevent circulatory overload. • Ritodrine decreases intensity and frequency of uterine contractions. • Don't use if solution is discolored or contains precipitate.

Oxytocin calculation

Your patient is 10 days overdue, so the doctor prescribes oxytocin to stimulate labor. The order reads *1 ml (10 U) oxytocin in 1 L (1,000 ml) NSS; infuse via pump at 2 mU/minute for 20 minutes, then increase flow rate to 3 mU/minute.* What is the solution's concentration? What is the flow rate needed to deliver 2 mU/minute for 20 minutes? What is the flow rate needed to deliver 3 mU/minute thereafter?

• Determine the concentration of the solution by setting up a proportion with the ordered concentration in one fraction and the unknown concentration in the other fraction:

$$\frac{10\,U}{1,000\,ml} = \frac{X\,U}{1\,ml}$$

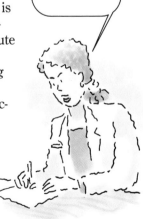

First, I determine the concentration of the solution.

• Cross-multiply the fractions:

$$X\,\text{U} \times 1{,}000\ \text{ml} = 10\,\text{U} \times 1\ \text{ml}$$

• Solve for X by dividing both sides of the equation by 1,000 ml and canceling units that appear in both the numerator and denominator:

$$\frac{X\,\text{U} \times \cancel{1{,}000\ \text{ml}}}{\cancel{1{,}000\ \text{ml}}} = \frac{10\,\text{U} \times 1\ \cancel{\text{ml}}}{1{,}000\ \cancel{\text{ml}}}$$

$$X = \frac{10\,\text{U}}{1{,}000}$$

$$X = 0.01\ \text{U}$$

• The amount 0.01 U can be written in milliunits (mU): 1 mU is $\frac{1}{1000}$ of a unit; 1,000 mU is 1 U. Therefore 0.01 U times 1,000 equals 10 mU. So, the concentration is 10 mU/ml.
• Next, determine the flow rate. If the prescribed dosage of oxytocin is 2 mU/minute for 20 minutes, the patient receives a total of 40 mU. To calculate the flow rate needed to provide that dose, set up the following proportion with the known concentration in one fraction and the total oxytocin dose and the unknown flow rate in the other fraction:

Before you give that drug

Learn from labels

Labels provide important information for calculating dosages. For example, examine the Pitocin label shown here.

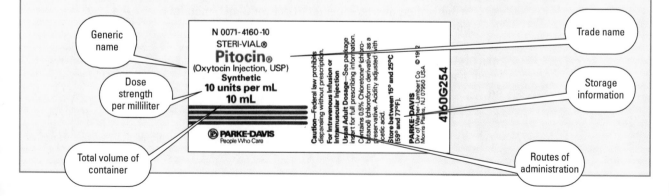

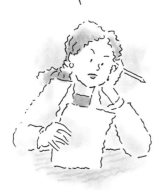

Next,
I determine
the flow rate
for the first
20 minutes.

$$\frac{10 \text{ mU}}{1 \text{ ml}} = \frac{40 \text{ mU}}{X \text{ ml}}$$

• Cross-multiply the fractions:

$$X \text{ ml} \times 10 \text{ mU} = 1 \text{ ml} \times 40 \text{ mU}$$

• Solve for X by dividing both sides of the equation by 10 mU and canceling units that appear in both the numerator and denominator:

$$\frac{X \text{ ml} \times \cancel{10 \text{ mU}}}{\cancel{10 \text{ mU}}} = \frac{1 \text{ ml} \times 40 \cancel{\text{ mU}}}{10 \cancel{\text{ mU}}}$$

$$X = \frac{40 \text{ ml}}{10}$$

$$X = 4 \text{ ml}$$

• The flow rate is 4 ml/20 minutes. Because this drug must be delivered by infusion pump, compute the hourly flow rate by multiplying the 20-minute rate by 3:

$$4 \text{ ml/20 minutes} \times 3 = 12 \text{ ml/hour}$$

• The hourly flow rate is 12 ml/hour. Finally, calculate the flow rate to be used after the first 20 minutes, to provide 3 mU/minute (180 mU/hour). Having calculated the solution's concentration as 10 mU/ml, set up the following proportion with the known concentration in one fraction and the increased oxytocin dose and the unknown flow rate in the other fraction:

Now
I determine
the flow rate
to be used after
the first
20 minutes.

$$\frac{10 \text{ mU}}{1 \text{ ml}} = \frac{180 \text{ mU}}{X \text{ ml}}$$

• Cross-multiply the fractions:

$$X \text{ ml} \times 10 \text{ mU} = 1 \text{ ml} \times 180 \text{ mU}$$

• Solve for X by dividing both sides of the equation by 10 mU and canceling units that appear in both the numerator and denominator:

$$\frac{X \text{ ml} \times \cancel{10 \text{ mU}}}{\cancel{10 \text{ mU}}} = \frac{1 \text{ ml} \times 180 \cancel{\text{ mU}}}{10 \cancel{\text{ mU}}}$$

$$X = \frac{180 \text{ ml}}{10}$$

$$X = 18 \text{ ml}$$

• After 20 minutes, reset the pump to deliver 18 ml/hour. That's 18 ml/60 minutes, or 0.3 ml/minute. Because there are 10 mU/ml, multiply 10 by 0.3 ml/minute to verify that this flow rate does provide 3 mU/minute.

Seizure prevention

Your patient had a seizure due to pregnancy-induced hypertension. The doctor orders *4 g (4,000 mg) of magnesium sulfate in 250 ml D₅W to be infused at 2 g/hour.* What is the flow rate in milliliters per hour?

There are two approaches to solving this problem.

Concentration and flow approach

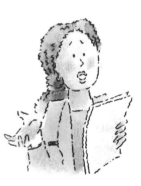

• One way to approach this problem is to set up a proportion with the known concentration in one fraction and the flow rate in grams and the unknown flow rate in milliliters in the other fraction:

$$\frac{4\text{ g}}{250\text{ ml}} = \frac{2\text{ g}}{X\text{ ml}}$$

• Cross-multiply the fractions:

$$X\text{ ml} \times 4\text{ g} = 250\text{ ml} \times 2\text{ g}$$

• Solve for *X* by dividing each side of the equation by 4 g and canceling units that appear in both the numerator and denominator:

$$\frac{X\text{ ml} \times 4\cancel{\text{ g}}}{4\cancel{\text{ g}}} = \frac{250\text{ ml} \times 2\cancel{\text{ g}}}{4\cancel{\text{ g}}}$$

$$X = \frac{250\text{ ml} \times 2}{4}$$

$$X = \frac{500\text{ ml}}{4}$$

$$X = 125\text{ ml}$$

The magnesium sulfate solution should be infused at 125 ml/hour.

Strength and flow approach

• Another approach is to first calculate the strength of the solution by setting up a proportion with the known strength in one fraction and the unknown strength in the other fraction:

$$\frac{4\text{ g}}{250\text{ ml}} = \frac{X\text{ g}}{1\text{ ml}}$$

• Cross-multiply the fractions:

$$X\text{ g} \times 250\text{ ml} = 4\text{ g} \times 1\text{ ml}$$

• Solve for X by dividing each side of the equation by 250 ml and canceling units that appear in both the numerator and denominator:

$$\frac{X\text{ g} \times \cancel{250\text{ ml}}}{\cancel{250\text{ ml}}} = \frac{4\text{ g} \times 1\cancel{\text{ ml}}}{250\cancel{\text{ ml}}}$$

$$X = \frac{4\text{ g}}{250}$$

$$X = 0.016\text{ g}$$

• The solution's strength is 0.016 g/ml. Next, calculate the flow rate by setting up another proportion with the solution concentration in one fraction and the unknown flow rate in the other fraction:

$$\frac{X\text{ ml}}{2\text{ g}} = \frac{1\text{ ml}}{0.016\text{ g}}$$

• Cross-multiply the fractions:

$$X\text{ ml} \times 0.016\text{ g} = 1\text{ ml} \times 2\text{ g}$$

• Solve for X by dividing each side of the equation by 0.016 g and canceling units that appear in both the numerator and denominator:

$$\frac{X\text{ ml} \times \cancel{0.016\text{ g}}}{\cancel{0.016\text{ g}}} = \frac{1\text{ ml} \times 2\cancel{\text{ g}}}{0.016\cancel{\text{ g}}}$$

$$X = \frac{2\text{ ml}}{0.016}$$

$$X = 125\text{ ml}$$

The same flow rate of 125 ml per hour is obtained using this method.

Nothing feels better than getting the right answer twice!

Preterm labor prevention

Your patient is in preterm labor. The doctor prescribes *150 mg of ritodrine hydrochloride in 500 ml of D₅W to infuse at 0.35 mg/minute.* What is the flow rate for this solution?

• First, find the solution's strength. Set up the following proportion with the known strength in one fraction and the unknown strength in the other fraction:

$$\frac{X \text{ mg}}{1 \text{ ml}} = \frac{150 \text{ mg}}{500 \text{ ml}}$$

• Cross-multiply the fractions:

$$X \text{ mg} \times 500 \text{ ml} = 150 \text{ mg} \times 1 \text{ ml}$$

• Solve for X by dividing each side of the equation by 500 ml and canceling units that appear in both the numerator and denominator:

$$\frac{X \text{ mg} \times \cancel{500 \text{ ml}}}{\cancel{500 \text{ ml}}} = \frac{150 \text{ mg} \times 1 \cancel{\text{ ml}}}{500 \cancel{\text{ ml}}}$$

$$X = \frac{150 \text{ mg}}{500}$$

$$X = 0.3 \text{ mg}$$

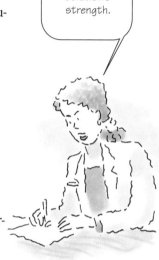

To begin, I calculate the solution's strength.

• The strength of the solution is 0.3 mg/ml. Next, calculate the flow rate needed to deliver the prescribed dose of 0.35 mg/minute. To do this, set up the following proportion with the known solution strength in one fraction and the unknown flow rate in the other fraction:

$$\frac{X \text{ ml}}{0.35 \text{ mg}} = \frac{1 \text{ ml}}{0.3 \text{ mg}}$$

• Cross-multiply the fractions:

$$X \text{ ml} \times 0.3 \text{ mg} = 1 \text{ ml} \times 0.35 \text{ mg}$$

• Solve for X by dividing each side of the equation by 0.3 mg and canceling units that appear in both the numerator and denominator:

$$\frac{X \text{ ml} \times \cancel{0.3 \text{ mg}}}{\cancel{0.3 \text{ mg}}} = \frac{1 \text{ ml} \times 0.35 \cancel{\text{ mg}}}{0.3 \cancel{\text{ mg}}}$$

$$X = 1.17 \text{ ml}$$

Then I calculate the flow rate per minute.

• The flow rate is 1.17 ml/minute. Because the infusion must be administered with a pump, compute the hourly flow rate by setting up a proportion with the flow rate per minute in one fraction and the unknown flow rate in the other fraction:

$$\frac{X \text{ ml}}{60 \text{ minutes}} = \frac{1.17 \text{ ml}}{1 \text{ minute}}$$

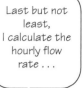

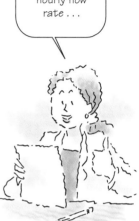

Last but not least,
I calculate the hourly flow rate . . .

• Cross-multiply the fractions:

$$X \text{ ml} \times 1 \text{ minute} = 1.17 \text{ ml} \times 60 \text{ minutes}$$

• Solve for X by dividing each side of the equation by 1 minute and canceling units that appear in both the numerator and denominator:

$$\frac{X \text{ ml} \times 1 \text{ minute}}{1 \text{ minute}} = \frac{1.17 \text{ ml} \times 60 \text{ minutes}}{1 \text{ minute}}$$

$$X = 70.2 \text{ ml}$$

Round off the answer to the nearest milliliter and set the infusion pump to deliver 70 ml/hour.

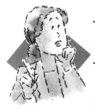

Quick quiz

1. If the order reads *150 mg of ritodrine in 1,000 ml of D_5W,* the solution's concentration is:
   A. 15 mg/ml
   B. 0.15 mg/ml
   C. 150 mg/ml

Answer: B. To solve this problem, set up a proportion with the known concentration in one fraction and the unknown concentration in the other fraction. Then solve for X.

2. A sudden increase or decrease in the fetal heart rate after drug treatment is:
   A. a sign that the infant is about to be delivered.
   B. a sign of an adverse reaction to the drug.
   C. a temporary reaction to many obstetric drugs.

Answer: B. If changes in the fetal heart rate occur, discontinue the drug immediately.

3. If an order says to *infuse 20 mg of terbutaline sulfate in 1,000 ml of D₅W at 0.01 mg/minute for 20 minutes,* the flow rate should be:

    A. 1 ml

    B. 10 ml

    C. 100 ml

Answer: B. First, calculate the concentration, which is 0.02 mg/ml. Then determine the amount of drug provided in 20 minutes by multiplying 0.01 by 20 minutes to get 0.2 mg. Finally, set up a proportion with the concentration in one fraction and the total amount of medication and the unknown flow rate in the other fraction. Solve for *X* to get 10 ml.

4. If 5 g of magnesium sulfate are added to 1 L of normal saline solution, the concentration of magnesium sulfate is:

    A. 5 mg/ml

    B. 50 mg/ml

    C. 0.05 mg/ml

Answer: A. First, convert 5 g to 5,000 mg and 1 L to 1,000 ml. Then divide the 1,000 into 5,000 to obtain the concentration of the solution: 5 mg/ml.

5. If the doctor orders *20 g of magnesium sulfate in 1,000 ml of D₅W to be infused at 5 g/hour,* the flow rate in milliliters per hour is:

    A. 2 ml/hour.

    B. 25 ml/hour.

    C. 250 ml/hour.

Answer: C. To solve this problem, set up a proportion with the ordered concentration in one fraction and the flow rate in grams and the unknown flow rate in milliliters in the other fraction. Solve for *X*.

Scoring

☆☆☆   If you answered all five items correctly, fantastic! Your labors have helped you become a confident calculator!

☆☆   If you answered four correctly, keep at it! You'll soon be able to deftly deliver drugs on any delivery unit!

☆   If you answered fewer than four correctly, don't worry! You still have one chapter left to conquer the Quick Quiz!

14

Calculating critical care dosages

Just the facts

In this chapter, you'll learn:

♦ special points to consider when giving critical care drugs

♦ how to calculate dosages for intravenous (I.V.) push drugs

♦ how to calculate I.V. flow rates for critical care drugs

♦ how to calculate drugs not ordered at a specific flow rate or dosage.

A look at critical care dosages

If you work on a critical care unit, you not only need to perform dosage calculations accurately, you also need to perform them quickly because of the patient's life-threatening condition. (See *Quick list of critical care meds and measurements*, page 268.)

Many I.V. drugs — such as the antiarrhythmics, lidocaine and bretylium; the vasodilators, sodium nitroprusside and nitroglycerin; and the adrenergics, norepinephrine and dopamine — are administered in life-threatening situations. The nurse's job is to prepare the drug for infusion, give it to the patient, and then observe him to evaluate the drug's effectiveness.

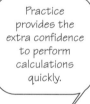

Practice provides the extra confidence to perform calculations quickly.

Administering I.V. injections

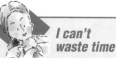

Many drugs administered on critical care units are given by direct injection, also called I.V. push. These potent, fast-acting drugs rapidly control heart rate, respirations, blood pressure, cardiac output, or kidney function. They usually have a short duration of action, so you can evaluate their effectiveness immediately and begin other treatment promptly if they're not working.

Quick list of critical care meds and measurements

The list below shows some common critical care drugs and associated units of measure. Memorizing these units of measure will help speed your calculations:

One critical difference

Generally, the doctor orders I.V. push drugs by flow rate (ml/hour or gtt/minute) or by dosage (mcg/kg/minute or mg/minute).

Calculate dosages on the critical care unit the same as you would on other units. However, take extra care because drugs used on critical care units are extremely potent and have serious adverse effects including death.

- epinephrine: mg/minute
- nitroglycerin: mg/minute
- norepinephrine: mcg/minute
- phenylephrine: mcg/minute
- nitroprusside: mcg/kg/minute
- dopamine: mcg/kg/minute
- dobutamine: mcg/kg/minute
- procainamide: mg/minute
- lidocaine: mg/minute.

One big responsibility

You're responsible for calculating and administering the dose accurately, following any special instructions. Many drugs used on critical care units come in small vials, so double-check the label to make sure you're giving the right dose or concentration. For example, epinephrine comes in two concentrations, 1:1,000 and 1:10,000. Giving the wrong concentration could be fatal.

Because calculating dosages during an emergency is stressful, and stress makes you more error-prone, do everything you can to be prepared. (See *Stress busters.*)

Calculating dosages

The following examples demonstrate how to use proportions to calculate I.V. push drugs. Note that the calculations are very similar to those for intramuscular drugs.

Also note how the administration times vary. If you're not sure how slowly or quickly to push a drug, look it up or call the pharmacist. It's better to be safe than sorry with rapid-acting drugs.

Look at the label

Your patient is admitted with frequent ventricular arrhythmias. The doctor orders *procainamide 200 mg q5mins by slow I.V. push (no faster than 25 to 50 mg/minute) until arrhythmias disappear.* If the drug label says to administer 100 mg/ml, how many milliliters of procainamide should you give to the patient every five minutes?

• Set up a proportion with the ordered dose and the unknown dose in one fraction and the dose in milligrams per milliliter in the other fraction:

$$\frac{200 \text{ mg}}{X \text{ ml}} = \frac{100 \text{ mg}}{1 \text{ ml}}$$

• Cross-multiply the fractions:

$$X \text{ ml} \times 100 \text{ mg} = 1 \text{ ml} \times 200 \text{ mg}$$

• Solve for X by dividing each side of the equation by 100 mg and canceling the units that appear in both the numerator and denominator:

$$\frac{X \text{ ml} \times \cancel{100 \text{ mg}}}{\cancel{100 \text{ mg}}} = \frac{1 \text{ ml} \times 200 \, \cancel{\text{mg}}}{100 \, \cancel{\text{mg}}}$$

$$X = 2 \text{ ml}$$

You should administer 2 ml, or one-fifth of the contents of the procainamide vial. According to the package insert, you should administer the drug only I.M. or I.V. Also note

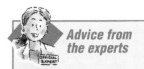

Advice from the experts

Stress busters

Here are four hot tips to help reduce your stress level when calculating drugs in an emergency:

• Carry a list of all the drug-calculation formulas.
• Carry a calculator for quick use.
• Convert your patients' weights to kilograms and keep the information at the bedside.
• Become familiar with the different critical care drugs given I.V.

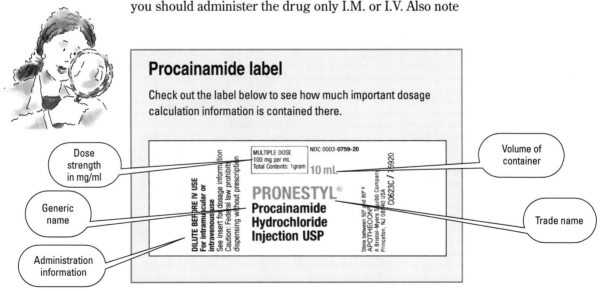

Procainamide label

Check out the label below to see how much important dosage calculation information is contained there.

Dose strength in mg/ml

Generic name

Administration information

MULTIPLE DOSE
100 mg per mL
Total Contents: 1gram

NDC 0003-0759-20

10 mL

DILUTE BEFORE IV USE
For intramuscular or
intravenous use
See insert for dosage information
Caution: Federal law prohibits
dispensing without prescription

PRONESTYL®
Procainamide
Hydrochloride
Injection USP

Store between 59° and 86° F
APOTHECON
A Bristol-Myers Squibb Company
Princeton, NJ 08540 USA

C0623C / 75920

Volume of container

Trade name

that when giving procainamide I.V., the drug must be diluted.

Rapid heartbeat riddle

Your patient suddenly develops supraventricular tachycardia. The doctor orders *6 mg of adenosine rapid I.V. push.* If the only vial available contains 3 mg/ml, how many milliliters should you give?

• Set up a proportion with the available solution in one ratio and the ordered dose and the unknown dose in the other ratio:

$$3 \text{ mg} : 1 \text{ ml} :: 6 \text{ mg} : X \text{ ml}$$

• Multiply the extremes and the means:

$$X \text{ ml} \times 3 \text{ mg} = 1 \text{ ml} \times 6 \text{ mg}$$

• Solve for X by dividing both sides of the equation by 3 mg and canceling units that appear in both the numerator and denominator:

$$\frac{X \text{ ml} \times \cancel{3 \text{ mg}}}{\cancel{3 \text{ mg}}} = \frac{1 \text{ ml} \times 6 \cancel{\text{mg}}}{3 \cancel{\text{mg}}}$$

$$X = \frac{6 \text{ ml}}{3}$$

$$X = 2 \text{ ml}$$

You should administer 2 ml of the solution. According to the package insert, this drug should be administered by rapid I.V. push due to its very short half-life. It also should be administered directly into the vein or in the most proximal port, followed by a rapid saline flush.

Digoxin difficulty

Your patient has a history of rapid atrial fibrillation and takes digoxin at home. When his digoxin level is found to be subtherapeutic, the doctor orders *0.125 mg of I.V digoxin as a single dose* to control his heart rate. The only available digoxin vial contains 0.25 mg/ml. How many milliliters should you give?

• Set up a proportion with the available solution in one ratio and the ordered dose and the unknown dose in the other ratio:

$$0.25 \text{ mg} : 1 \text{ ml} :: 0.125 \text{ mg} : X \text{ ml}$$

• Multiply the means and the extremes:

$$X \text{ ml} \times 0.25 \text{ mg} = 1 \text{ ml} \times 0.125 \text{ mg}$$

• Solve for X by dividing both sides of the equation by 0.25 mg and canceling units that appear in both the numerator and denominator:

$$\frac{X \text{ ml} \times \cancel{0.25 \text{ mg}}}{\cancel{0.25 \text{ mg}}} = \frac{1 \text{ ml} \times 0.125 \cancel{\text{ mg}}}{0.25 \cancel{\text{ mg}}}$$

$$X = 0.5 \text{ ml}$$

You should administer 0.5 ml of digoxin. According to the package insert, give it by I.V. push over 5 minutes.

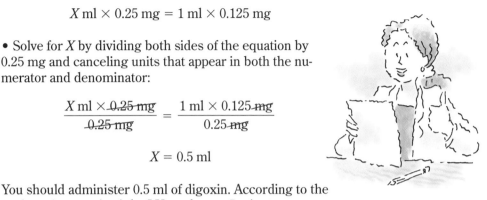

Calculating I.V. flow rates

Because many drugs given on the critical care unit are used to treat life-threatening problems, you can't waste time calculating I.V. flow rates. You must swiftly do the calculations, prepare the drug for infusion, administer it, and then observe the patient closely to evaluate the drug's effectiveness.

Three critical calculations

You may need to perform three calculations before administering critical care drugs:

1. concentration of the drug in the I.V. solution

2. flow rate required to deliver the desired dose

3. number of micrograms needed, based on the patient's weight in kilograms. You may need to perform this calculation if the drug is ordered in micrograms per kilogram of body weight per minute. *Remember: If you need to convert milligrams to micrograms, multiply by 1,000.*

Calculating concentration

To calculate the drug's concentration, use the following formula:

$$\text{concentration in mg/ml} = \frac{\text{mg of drug}}{\text{ml of fluid}}$$

• If you need to express the concentration in mcg/ml, multiply the answer by 1,000.

Figuring flow rate

You can determine the I.V. flow rate per minute, using the following formula:

> Use this formula to find the flow rate per minute . . .

$$\frac{\text{dose/minute}}{X\text{ ml/minute}} = \frac{\text{concentration of solution}}{1\text{ ml of fluid}}$$

• To calculate the hourly flow rate, first multiply the ordered dose, given in milligrams or micrograms per minute, by 60 minutes to determine the hourly dose. Then use the following proportion to compute the hourly flow rate:

> . . .and this one to find the hourly flow rate.

$$\frac{\text{hourly dose}}{X\text{ ml/hour}} = \frac{\text{concentration of solution}}{1\text{ ml of fluid}}$$

Determining the dosage

To determine the dosage in milligrams per kilogram of body weight per minute, perform the following steps:
• First, determine the concentration of the solution in milligrams per milliliter. To determine the dose in milligrams per hour, multiply the hourly flow rate by the concentration using the formula:

$$\text{dose in mg/hour} = \text{hourly flow rate} \times \text{concentration}$$

• To calculate the dose in milligrams per minute, first divide the hourly dose by 60 minutes.
   Here's the formula:

$$\text{dose in mg/minute} = \frac{\text{dose in mg/hour}}{60\text{ minutes}}$$

• Then divide the dose per minute by the patient's weight, using this formula:

$$\text{mg/kg/minute} = \frac{\text{mg/minute}}{\text{patient's weight in kg}}$$

• Once you've performed these calculations, make sure that the drug is being given within a safe and therapeutic range. Compare the amount in milligrams per kilogram per minute to the safe range shown in a drug reference book. (See *No time for books?*)

Real world problems

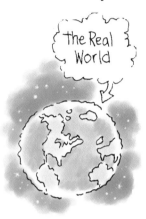

The following examples show how to calculate an I.V. flow rate using the different formulas.

Problem #1

Your patient is having frequent runs of ventricular tachycardia that subside after 10 to 12 beats. So the doctor orders *2 g (2,000 mg) of lidocaine in 500 ml of D₅W to infuse at 2 mg/minute.* What is the flow rate in milliliters per minute? In milliliters per hour?

• First, find the solution's concentration by setting up a proportion with the unknown concentration in one fraction and the ordered dose in the other fraction:

$$\frac{X \text{ mg}}{1 \text{ ml}} = \frac{2,000 \text{ mg}}{500 \text{ ml}}$$

• Cross-multiply the fractions:

$$X \text{ mg} \times 500 \text{ ml} = 2,000 \text{ mg} \times 1 \text{ ml}$$

• Solve for *X* by dividing each side of the equation by

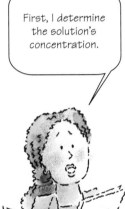

First, I determine the solution's concentration.

I can't waste time

No time for books?

Suppose you don't have time to refer to your dosage calculation book in a critical situation. Keep these formulas on a card with your calculator for quick reference. They're foolproof!

• To find out how many micrograms per kilogram per minute your patient is receiving, use this formula:

$$\frac{\text{mg}}{\text{volume of bag}} \times 1000 \div 60 \div \text{kg} \times \text{ infusion rate} = \text{mcg/kg/min}$$

• To find out how many milliliters per hour you should give, use this formula:

$$\frac{\text{weight in kg} \times \text{dose in mcg/kg/min} \times 60}{\text{concentration in 1L}} = \text{ml/hr}$$

500 ml and canceling units that appear in both the numerator and denominator:

$$\frac{X \text{ mg} \times \cancel{500 \text{ ml}}}{\cancel{500 \text{ ml}}} = \frac{2,000 \text{ mg} \times 1 \cancel{\text{ml}}}{500 \cancel{\text{ml}}}$$

$$X = \frac{2,000 \text{ mg}}{500}$$

$$X = 4 \text{ mg}$$

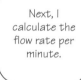

Next, I
calculate the
flow rate per
minute.

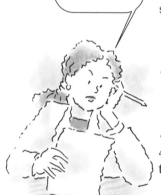

• The solution's concentration is 4 mg/ml. Next, calculate
the flow rate per minute needed to deliver the ordered
dose of 2 mg/minute. To do this, set up a proportion with
the unknown flow rate per minute in one fraction and the
solution's concentration in the other fraction:

$$\frac{2 \text{ mg}}{X \text{ ml}} = \frac{4 \text{ mg}}{1 \text{ ml}}$$

• Cross-multiply the fractions:

$$X \text{ ml} \times 4 \text{ mg} = 1 \text{ ml} \times 2 \text{ mg}$$

• Solve for X by dividing each side of the equation by
4 mg and canceling units that appear in both the numerator and denominator:

$$\frac{X \text{ ml} \times \cancel{4 \text{ mg}}}{\cancel{4 \text{ mg}}} = \frac{1 \text{ ml} \times 2 \cancel{\text{mg}}}{4 \cancel{\text{mg}}}$$

$$X = \frac{2 \text{ ml}}{4}$$

$$X = 0.5 \text{ ml}$$

Finally,
I calculate
the hourly flow
rate.

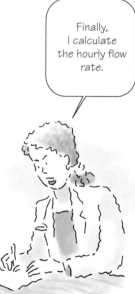

• The patient should receive 0.5 ml/minute of lidocaine.
Because lidocaine must be infused through an infusion
pump, compute the hourly flow rate. Do this by setting up
a proportion with the unknown flow rate per hour in one
fraction and the flow rate per minute in the other fraction:

$$\frac{X \text{ ml}}{60 \text{ minutes}} = \frac{0.5 \text{ ml}}{1 \text{ minute}}$$

• Cross-multiply the fractions:

$$X \text{ ml} \times 1 \text{ minute} = 0.5 \text{ ml} \times 60 \text{ minutes}$$

• Solve for X by dividing each side of the equation by 1 minute and canceling units that appear in both the numerator and denominator:

$$\frac{X \text{ ml} \times \cancel{1 \text{ minute}}}{\cancel{1 \text{ minute}}} = \frac{0.5 \text{ ml} \times 60 \cancel{\text{ minutes}}}{1 \cancel{\text{ minute}}}$$

$$X = 30 \text{ ml}$$

Set the infusion pump to deliver 30 ml/hour.

Problem #2

A 200-lb patient is to receive an I.V. infusion of dobutamine at 10 mcg/kg/minute. The label says to check the package insert. There it says to dilute 250 mg of the drug in 50 ml of D$_5$W. (See *Dobutamine label*.)

Because the drug vial contains 20 ml of solution, the total to be infused is 70 ml (50 ml of D$_5$W + 20 ml of solution). The solution's concentration is 3.6 mg/ml. How many milliliters of the drug should the patient receive each minute? Each hour?

• First, compute the patient's weight in kilograms. To do this, set up a proportion with the weight in pounds and the unknown weight in kilograms in one fraction and the number of pounds per kilogram in the other fraction:

$$\frac{200 \text{ lb}}{X \text{ kg}} = \frac{2.2 \text{ lb}}{1 \text{ kg}}$$

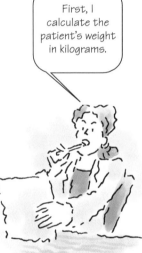

First, I calculate the patient's weight in kilograms.

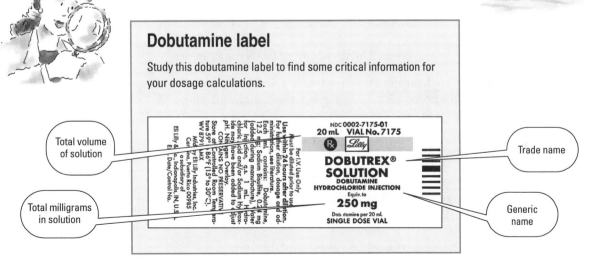

Dobutamine label

Study this dobutamine label to find some critical information for your dosage calculations.

Total volume of solution

Total milligrams in solution

NDC 0002-7175-01
20 mL   VIAL No. 7175

℞   *Lilly*

**DOBUTREX®
SOLUTION**
DOBUTAMINE
HYDROCHLORIDE INJECTION
Equiv. to
250 mg
Dob itamine per 20 mL
SINGLE DOSE VIAL

Trade name

Generic name

• Cross-multiply the fractions:

$$X \text{ kg} \times 2.2 \text{ lb} = 1 \text{ kg} \times 200 \text{ lb}$$

• Solve for X by dividing each side of the equation by 2.2 lb and canceling units that appear in both the numerator and denominator:

$$\frac{X \text{ kg} \times \cancel{2.2 \text{ lb}}}{\cancel{2.2 \text{ lb}}} = \frac{1 \text{ kg} \times 200 \cancel{\text{ lb}}}{2.2 \cancel{\text{ lb}}}$$

$$X = \frac{200 \text{ kg}}{2.2}$$

$$X = 90.9 \text{ kg}$$

• The patient weighs 90.9 kg. Next, determine the dose in micrograms per minute by setting up a proportion with the patient's weight in kilograms and the unknown dose in micrograms per minute in one fraction and the known dose in micrograms per kilogram per minute in the other fraction:

$$\frac{90.9 \text{ kg}}{X \text{ mcg/minute}} = \frac{1 \text{ kg}}{10 \text{ mcg/minute}}$$

• Cross-multiply the fractions:

$$X \text{ mcg/minute} \times 1 \text{ kg} = 10 \text{ mcg/minute} \times 90.9 \text{ kg}$$

• Solve for X by dividing each side of the equation by 1 kg and canceling units that appear in both the numerator and denominator:

$$\frac{X \text{ mcg/minute} \times \cancel{1 \text{ kg}}}{\cancel{1 \text{ kg}}} = \frac{10 \text{ mcg/minute} \times 90.9 \cancel{\text{ kg}}}{1 \cancel{\text{ kg}}}$$

$$X = 909 \text{ mcg/minute or } 0.909 \text{ mg/minute.}$$

• To determine the flow rate in milliliters per minute, set up a proportion using the solution's concentration and solve for X:

$$\frac{0.909 \text{ mg}}{X \text{ ml}} = \frac{3.6 \text{ mg}}{1 \text{ ml}}$$

$$X = 0.2525 \text{ ml/minute.}$$

• To find the flow rate in milliliters per hour, multiply by 60.

$$0.2525 \text{ ml/minute} \times 60 \text{ minutes/hour} = 15.15 \text{ ml/hour.}$$

The patient should receive 15 ml/hr.

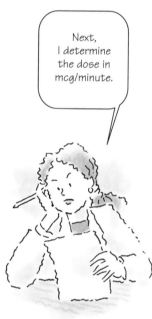

Next, I determine the dose in mcg/minute.

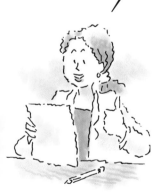

Finally, I calculate the dose in ml/hour.

Special cases

Critical care drugs aren't always ordered at a specific flow rate or dosage. Sometimes, they're prescribed according to the patient's heart rate, blood pressure, or other parameters.

In some cases, the doctor may order a starting dose and a maximum dose to which the drug can be titrated. To deliver the correct amount of drug, you must calculate the starting dose and the maximum dose.

Here are some examples of drug calculations that you may use in special cases.

Nipride number cruncher

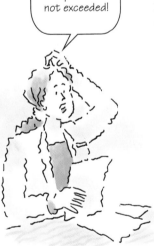

In this case, I have to make sure the maximum dose for this patient is not exceeded!

A patient with severe hypertension weighs 85 kg. The doctor's order reads *nipride 50 mg in 250 ml of D_5W. Start at 0.5 mcg/kg/minute. Titrate to keep systolic BP < 170 mm Hg. Maximum dose is 5 mcg/kg/minute.* How many micrograms per minute should the patient receive?

• Set up a proportion with the patient's weight and the unknown dose per minute in one fraction and the starting dose per minute in the other fraction:

$$\frac{85 \text{ kg}}{X \text{ mcg}} = \frac{1 \text{ kg}}{0.5 \text{ mcg}}$$

• Cross-multiply the fractions:

$$X \text{ mcg} \times 1 \text{ kg} = 0.5 \text{ mcg} \times 85 \text{ kg}$$

• Solve for X by dividing each side of the equation by 1 kg and canceling units that appear in both the numerator and denominator:

$$\frac{X \text{ mcg} \times \cancel{1 \text{ kg}}}{\cancel{1 \text{ kg}}} = \frac{0.5 \text{ mcg} \times 85 \cancel{\text{ kg}}}{1 \cancel{\text{ kg}}}$$

$$X = 42.5 \text{ mcg}$$

The starting dose is 42.5 mcg/minute.

How much phenylephrine in saline?

A patient with terminal Hodgkin's disease who weighs 90 lb (41 kg) has been hypotensive for several hours despite receiving I.V. fluid boluses. The doctor orders

100 mg of phenylephrine in 250 ml of normal saline solution. The drug is to start at 30 mcg/minute and then be titrated to keep the systolic blood pressure at 90 mm Hg. What is the flow rate in milliliters per minute?

First, I determine the concentration.

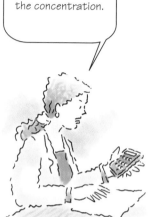

• First, determine the solution's concentration by dividing the ordered dose of phenylephrine by the amount of normal saline solution:

$$X = \frac{100\ mg}{250\ ml}$$

$$X = 0.4\ mg/ml$$

• The concentration is 0.4 mg/ml. Next, convert milligrams to micrograms by multiplying by 1,000:

$$0.4\ mg/ml \times 1,000 = 400\ mcg/ml$$

Next, I convert milligrams to micrograms.

• The concentration is 400 mcg/ml. Now, calculate the flow rate by setting up a proportion with the starting flow rate and the unknown flow rate in one fraction and the concentration in the other fraction:

$$\frac{30\ mcg/minute}{X\ ml/minute} = \frac{400\ mcg}{1\ ml}$$

• Cross-multiply the fractions:

$$X\ ml/minute \times 400\ mcg = 30\ mcg/minute \times 1\ ml$$

Finally, I find the hourly flow rate!

• Solve for *X* by dividing each side of the equation by 400 mcg and canceling units that appear in both the numerator and denominator:

$$\frac{X\ ml/minute \times \cancel{400\ mcg}}{\cancel{400\ mcg}} = \frac{30\ \cancel{mcg}/minute \times 1\ ml}{400\ \cancel{mcg}}$$

$$X = \frac{30\ ml/minute}{400}$$

$$X = 0.075\ ml/minute$$

• The flow rate is 0.075 ml/minute. To calculate the hourly flow rate, multiply 0.075 ml by 60:

$$0.075\ ml \times 60 = 4.5\ ml$$

The hourly flow rate is 4.5 ml rounded off to 5 ml/hour.

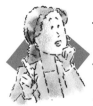

Quick quiz

1. If a patient has a dopamine drip of 800 mg in 500 ml of D_5W, the concentration is:
  A. 0.16 mg/ml
  B. 1.6 mg/ml
  C. 160 mg/ml

Answer: B. Concentration is determined by dividing the total in milligrams (800 mg) by the volume (500 ml).

2. Procainamide is measured in:
  A. mcg/kg/minute.
  B. mg/minute.
  C. mg/hour.

Answer: B. This information is necessary before you can calculate dosages of procainamide.

3. To convert milligrams to micrograms, multiply by:
  A. 60
  B. 10
  C. 1,000

Answer: C. When converting a number from milligrams to micrograms, move the decimal three spaces to the right.

4. How many kilograms does a 250-lb man weigh?
  A. 114 kg
  B. 11.4 kg
  C. 550 kg

Answer: A. To convert pounds to kilograms, divide by 2.2 and round off the number.

5. The doctor's order reads *Lasix 80 mg I.V. as a single dose.* The available vial contains 100 mg in 10 ml of normal saline solution. What volume should you give to accomplish this dose?
  A. 0.8 ml
  B. 8 ml
  C. 0.08 ml

Answer: B. Set up a proportion with the available solution in one ratio and the ordered dose and the unknown volume in the other ratio. Solve for *X*.

6. If a patient weighs 50 kg, his weight in pounds is:
   A.   110 lb
   B.   200 lb
   C.   28 lb

Answer: A. To convert kilograms to pounds multiply by 2.2.

Scoring

☆☆☆   If you answered all six items correctly, fantastic! You can calculate confidently in critical cases!

☆☆   If you answered five correctly, that's not bad! You're a cool, calm, and collected calculator!

☆   If you answered fewer than five correctly, don't fret! You have the best dosage calc book ever! Keep it with you always and refer to it frequently.

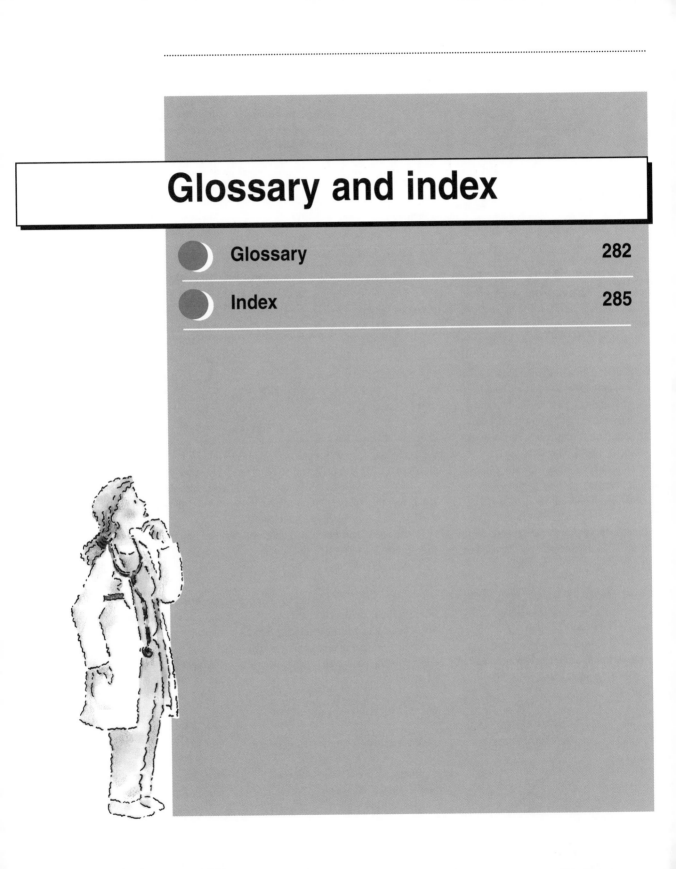

Glossary and index

Glossary

Apothecaries' system: measurement system used to measure liquid volumes and solid weights based on the units drop, minim, and grain, with amounts expressed in Roman numerals; used before the metric system became established

Avoirdupois system: measurement system used for ordering certain pharmaceutical products and for weighing patients; based on the units grain, ounce, and pound

body surface area (BSA): the area covered by a person's external skin calculated in square meters (m^2) according to height and weight; used to calculate safe pediatric dosages for all drugs and to calculate safe dosages for adult patients receiving extremely potent drugs or drugs requiring great precision, such as antineoplastic or chemotherapeutic agents

Clark's rule: equation used to verify drug dosages for children over age 2; based on weight

common factor: a number that is a factor of two different numbers (For example, 2 is a common factor of 4 and 6.)

common fraction: fraction with a whole number in numerator and denominator such as $\frac{2}{3}$

complex fraction: fraction in which numerator and denominator also are fractions such as:

$$\frac{2/7}{5/16}$$

concentration: ratio that expresses the amount of a drug in solution; sometimes called drug strength

denominator: the bottom number in a fraction, which represents the total number of equal parts of a whole; as opposed to the top number, or numerator, which represents the number of parts being considered (For example, in the fraction $\frac{7}{10}$, the denominator is 10.)

dividend: in division, the number to be divided (For example, in the problem $33 \div 7$, 33 is the dividend.)

divisor: in division, the number by which the dividend is divided (For example, in the problem $33 \div 7$, 7 is the divisor.)

drip factor: the number of drops calibrated to be delivered per milliliter of solution in an I.V. administration set, measured in gtt/ml (drops per milliliter); listed on the package containing the I.V. tubing administration set

drip rate: the number of drops of I.V. solution to be infused per minute; based on the drip factor (number of drops delivered per millimeter) and calibrated for the selected I.V. tubing

enteral: pertaining to the small intestine

equianalgesic dose: amount of a narcotic that provides the same pain relief as 10 mg of intramuscular (I.M) morphine; used to recalculate the necessary dose when substituting one analgesic for another

flow rate: the number of milliliters of I.V. fluid to administer over 1 hour, based on the total volume to be infused in milliliters and the amount of time for the infusion

fraction: representation of the division of one number by another number; mathematical expression for parts of a whole, with the bottom number (denominator) describing the total number of parts and the top number (numerator) describing the parts of the whole being considered; for example, $\frac{1}{2}$, $\frac{1}{3}$, $\frac{7}{18}$

Fried's rule: equation used to verify drug dosages for infants under age 1; based on age

glucometer: device used to calculate blood glucose levels — and, thereby, insulin levels — from a drop of blood

gram (g): basic unit of weight in the metric system; represents the weight of one cubic centimeter of water at 4° C

household system: measurement system that uses familiar household items, such as teaspoons, to measure drugs

improper fraction: fraction in which numerator is larger than or equal to the denominator, such as $\frac{3}{2}$, $\frac{10}{7}$, and $\frac{5}{5}$

International System of Units: system adopted in 1960 by the International Bureau of Weights and Measures to promote use of standard metric abbreviations to prevent drug transcription errors

largest common divisor: in a fraction the largest whole number that can be divided into both the numerator and denominator (For example, in the fraction $^8/_{10}$, the largest common divisor is 2.)

liter (L): basic unit of fluid volume in the metric system; equivalent to $^1/_{10}$ of a cubic meter

lowest common denominator: smallest number that's a multiple of all denominators in a set of fractions; also called least common multiple (For example, for the fractions, $^1/_{100}$ and $^3/_{150}$, the lowest common denominator is 300.)

lowest terms: in a fraction, the smallest numbers possible in the numerator and denominator (Reduce a fraction to its lowest terms by dividing the numerator and denominator by the largest common divisor. For example, in the fraction $^3/_{15}$, divide both the numerator and denominator by 3, the largest common divisor, to find $^1/_5$, the lowest terms of this fraction.)

meter (m): basic unit of length in the metric system; equivalent to 39.27 inches

metric system: decimal-based measurement system that uses the units meter (for length), liter (for volume), and gram (for weight); most widely used system for measuring amounts of drugs

milliequivalent (mEq): number of grams of a solute in 1 ml of normal solution; used to measure electrolytes

mixed number: number that consists of a whole number and a fraction, such as $1^1/_2$

multiplied common denominator: for a set of fractions, the product of all the denominators, which is found by multiplying all the denominators together (For example, for the fractions, $^1/_2$, $^2/_3$, and $^3/_5$, multiply the denominators together to find the multiplied common denominator, which is 30 $[2 \times 3 \times 5 = 30]$.)

nonparenteral drugs: drugs administered by the oral, topical, or rectal route, as opposed to drugs administered by the parenteral route

nomogram: chart used to determine body surface area in square meters, based on the patient's height and weight

numerator: the top number in a fraction, which represents the number of parts being considered, as opposed to the bottom number, the denominator, which represents the total number of equal parts of the whole (For example, in the fraction $^7/_{10}$, the numerator is 7.)

oral route (P.O.): drug administration through the mouth

parenteral route: drug administration through a route other than the digestive tract, such as I.V., I.M., or S.C. injection

percentage: a quantity stated as a part per hundred; written with a percent sign (%), which means "for every hundred" (For example, 50% represents 50 parts out of 100 total parts.)

prime factor: prime numbers that can be divided into some part of a mathematical expression such as the denominators in a set of fractions; used to find the lowest common denominator for a set of fractions (For example, the prime factors for the denominators in the fractions $^1/_{10}$ and $^2/_3$ are 5, 2, and 3.)

prime number: whole number that's evenly divisible only by 1 and itself, such as 2, 3, 5, and 7

product: the answer in multiplication (For example, in the equation, $4 \times 5 = 20$, the product is 20.)

proper fraction: fraction with a numerator that's smaller than the denominator such as $^1/_2$

proportion: set of equivalent ratios or fractions (An example of a proportion expressed by ratios is 2 : 3 :: 8 : 12, which is read as, "2 is to 3 as 8 is to 12." The same proportion expressed with fractions is $^2/_3 = {}^8/_{12}$.)

quotient: the answer in division (For example, in the equation $20 \div 5 = 4$, the quotient is 4.)

ratio: numerical way to compare items or show a relationship between numbers, with numbers separated by a colon, which represents the words, "is to" (For example, the ratio 4 : 5 is read as "4 is to 5." Ratios are commonly used to describe the relative proportions of ingredients such as the amount of drug relative to its solution.)

reciprocal: inverted fraction; used when dividing fractions (For example to divide $^1/_2$ by $^2/_3$, multiply $^1/_2$ by the reciprocal of $^2/_3$, which is $^3/_2$: in other words, $^1/_2 \div ^2/_3 = ^1/_2 \times ^3/_2 = ^3/_4$. When a fraction is multiplied by its reciprocal, the product is 1; for example, the reciprocal of the fraction $^2/_3$ is $^3/_2$, and $^2/_3 \times ^3/_2 = ^6/_6$ or 1.)

rectal route (P.R.): drug administration (usually by suppository) through the rectum

reduce: to simplify a numerical expression

by using the lowest possible numbers —
or lowest terms — to describe it (For
example, the fraction $^{15}/_{45}$ may be
reduced to $^1/_3$.)

rounding off: reducing the number of decimal places used to express a number (For
example, a decimal fraction that's expressed in thousandths may be rounded off
to the nearest hundredths or tenths; the
number 12.827 rounded off to the nearest
hundredths is 12.83. The same number
rounded off to the nearest tenths is 12.8.)

topical route: drug administration through
the skin, usually in cream, ointment, or
transdermal patch form; with application
of drug to the skin and absorption through
its layers into the circulation

transcribe: to write or type a copy of something; to record information by hand, tape-
recorder, or computer

unit system: measurement system that
expresses amount of a drug in units (U),
United States Pharmacopeia (USP) units,
or International Units (IU) (Drugs measured
in units include insulin, heparin, the topical
antibiotic bacitracin, and penicillin G and V.
Some forms of vitamin A and D are measured in USP units. The hormone calcitonin
and the fat-soluble vitamins A, D, and E are
measured in IUs.)

Young's rule: equation used to verify drug
dosages for children ages 2 to 12; based on
age

Index

i refers to an illustration; t refers to a table

i refers to an illustration; t refers to a table

i refers to an illustration; t refers to a table

i refers to an illustration; t refers to a table

i refers to an illustration; t refers to a table

i refers to an illustration; t refers to a table

i refers to an illustration; t refers to a table

W

Weight per volume solution, determining
       contents of, 180, 180t, 181, 181t
Whole, parts of, 2
Whole-number divisors, 29-30
Whole numbers, changing, into fraction, 53

X

X, finding value of, 50-65
    in common-fraction equations, 50-53
    in decimal-fraction equations, 54-56
    in proportion problems with fractions,
       59-61
    in proportion problems with ratios, 56-59
    metric unit conversion and, 76-77

Y

Young's rule, pediatric dosage verification
      and, 243
Yutopar, 254, 259t

Z

Zeros, adding or deleting, 27-28

i refers to an illustration; t refers to a table

Notes

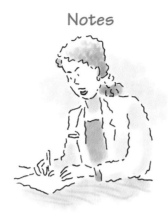

Notes

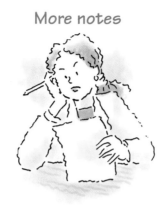

More notes

Still more notes

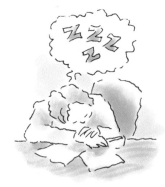